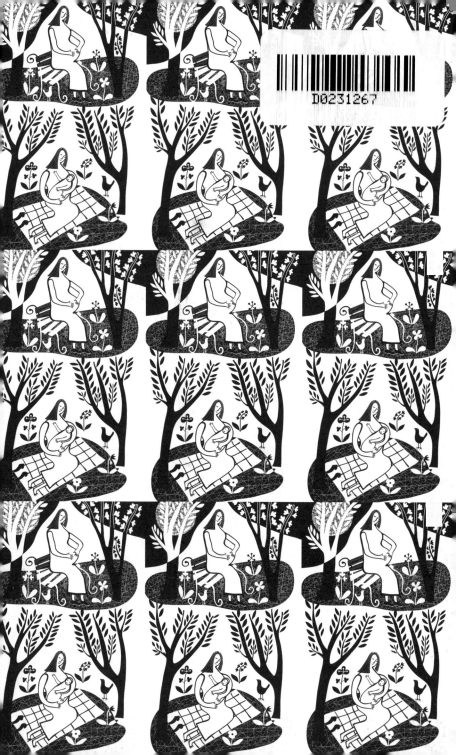

'This wonderful book is a must. Riga's style makes you feel like you're sharing a pot of tea by the fire, as she takes you through the stages of the childbearing year with grounded, accessible and simple mindfulness practices. *Mindful Pregnancy and Birth* is a warm invitation to all mothers-to-be to step into a circle of trust and faith with a calm mind and body, joyfully preparing for the changes ahead. This book will make your heart sing.'

KATE WOODS
CONSCIOUS BIRTHING INTERNATIONAL

'I love this book – so much needed in today's world when pregnant women are generally so stressed and unable to find an oasis to simply be with the pregnancy and the changes they are experiencing. There is no time more important to slow down, to find some silence and space within and develop the art of relaxation. This book will show you how easy and indeed natural it is to be mindful and how much that can change the quality of your life. You will find that you have time to connect with your unborn baby and communicate more meaningfully with your loved ones, without diminishing your ability to "do" things. When the mind is relaxed, the body follows suit. Then nature's plan for birth and loving connection can unfold in all its magnificence.
Read this book – it's life changing!'

JANET BALASKAS
AUTHOR OF 'NEW ACTIVE BIRTH'

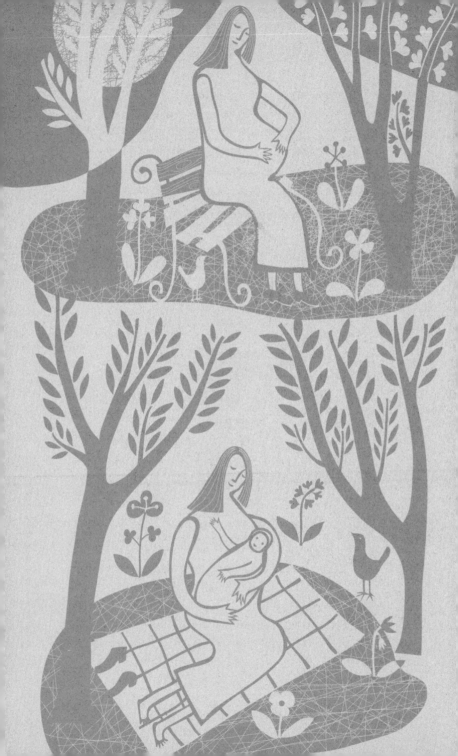

Mindful
Pregnancy & Birth

Nurturing Love and Awareness

Riga Forbes

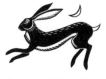

Leaping Hare Press

First published in the UK in 2017 by

Leaping Hare Press

An imprint of The Quarto Group
The Old Brewery, 6 Blundell Street
London N7 9BH, United Kingdom
T (0)20 7700 6700 **F** (0)20 7700 8066
www.quartoknows.com

Text © 2017 Riga Forbes
Design and layout © 2017 Quarto Publishing plc

British Library Cataloguing-in-Publication Data
A catalogue record for this book is available from the
British Library

ISBN: 978-1-78240-505-4

This book was conceived, designed and produced by

Leaping Hare Press

58 West Street, Brighton BN1 2RA, United Kingdom
Publisher SUSAN KELLY
Creative Director MICHAEL WHITEHEAD
Art Director JAMES LAWRENCE
Editorial Director TOM KITCH
Commissioning Editor MONICA PERDONI
Project Editor JOANNA BENTLEY
Designer GINNY ZEAL
Illustrator MELVYN EVANS

Printed in China

1 3 5 7 9 10 8 6 4 2

CONTENTS

Introduction 6

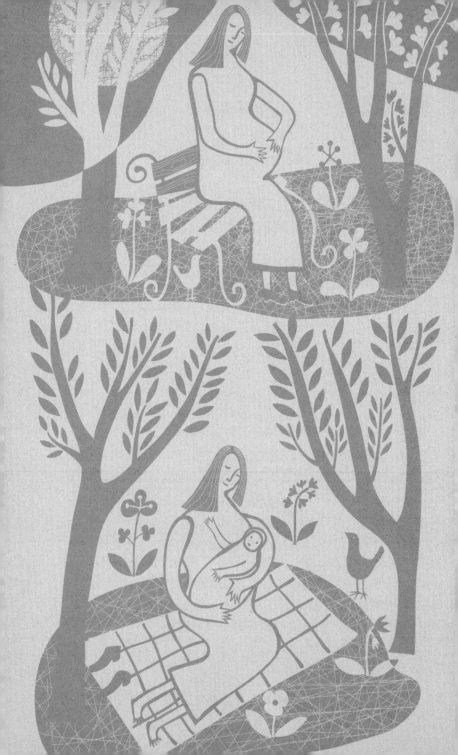

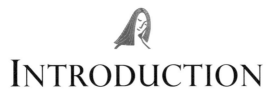

INTRODUCTION

*Pregnancy, birth and becoming a parent
are human rites of passage. For women, the
route into motherhood asks that we are physically
and emotionally able to surrender and to meet the
euphoria, endurance and all the in-betweens it will
bring. A father or co-parent will also find themselves
exploring new edges of their experience while
supporting their partner through birth and in
parenting their new baby. And, of course, this special
process will bring a beloved new life into being.
Building a foundation of mindfulness offers us
a core of stability as we make the transition
into parenthood.*

WHY PRACTISE
MINDFULNESS IN PREGNANCY?

◆

Life can be stressful. Yet in pregnancy, a woman needs intervals of regular relaxation to facilitate her body's intensive work of baby-making. As she approaches birth, she is physiologically primed by her hormones for this momentous event, and this too requires that she is relaxed. Meditation can become her courageous opportunity for deep relaxation.

MANY OF US HAVE RELENTLESSLY busy lifestyles, and the idea of slowing down or switching off from our constant schedules or the flood of stimuli around us can actually be scary. Fears of boredom or of losing our threads of connection to modern life might be daunting. And perhaps we'd just rather be busy – because if we weren't, then what would we be? If we were not identifying with our thinking mind, then who would we be?

The practice of mindfulness is not alluring to the mind that seeks to be busy, yet gradually and incrementally it can begin to show us a little more about the relationship between *ourselves* and our *thoughts*. Because they are not inseparable. In this way it is a remarkable resource, because as we practise, not only do we start to receive the nourishment of deep relaxation, but we also learn how to notice our thinking processes, rather than simply following and believing them.

And somewhere along the line it also activates the possibility of our minds becoming less busy, allowing us to give more of our full attention to our lives as they are, in this present moment – so that we can truly live them.

A Work of Art in Progress

Emotionally, pregnancy can be an intense time too, and having a quiet space to witness our feelings, to experience them as they are, without judging them or being overwhelmed, can also be very liberating. It can help us to feel calmer and more empowered and to develop compassion for ourselves, whatever state we are in. This approach could not be more needed or relevant than today, when pregnant women are managing full-time work and families, and the accumulated stress and tiredness in body and mind can have a detrimental effect on our overall well-being. We need to slow down in pregnancy in order to keep up with the work of art in progress inside us.

This is even more significant when we consider that stress has its roots in fear and that if we, as women, carry these responses and their associated hormones, such as adrenaline and cortisol, into the birth room, they can hinder our birthing process at a physiological level. What is especially important about keeping calm and maximizing positive emotions in labour is that firstly it makes the experience more comfortable, and even enjoyable, because the mind and therefore the body are able to relax and open more; secondly, it promotes the release of our key birthing hormones, which enable labour to progress steadily; and thirdly, it helps protect us from potentially stressful influences in our environment.

In very simple terms, relaxation is a woman's best birthing tool, and it will support her and her partner in so many ways throughout the entire perinatal year and beyond, into family life. By establishing a mindfulness practice, a mother can access her ability to relax more whenever she needs to, thereby reducing her own stress levels – because as we work with meditation, we not only address the physical tension in our bodies and our breathing, but we also develop more awareness of the inner realm of our thoughts and emotions, where stress is generated.

Labour of Love

Mindfulness practice can allow us to witness our inner narratives, trigger points, ideas and feelings, both positive and negative, in an unidentified way, so that we can observe these internal conversations and beliefs without reacting to them. So, for example, if we encounter inner thought processes that could lead us into a state of anxiety, it becomes possible for us to watch and listen to our experience without necessarily succumbing to our habitual cycle of stress-responses to it.

A pregnant woman can use this in pregnancy to alleviate fear she may be holding around the coming birth, just as she can use it in labour to reduce fear and discomfort and to let her body do its extraordinary work. This practice will also benefit a father, partner or birth partner by helping them to keep breathing, relaxing and staying present to the mother while supporting her to the best of their ability.

And if, as I believe, the path of having children is what we call 'a labour of love', then mindfulness also offers parents a portal through which compassion can enter and bring us back to our hearts when we have missed night after night of sleep. Because in the midst of this intensely beautiful and challenging first phase of parenthood, we become students of love, beginning with self-kindness, and in meditation we can cultivate an inner space for love to be present.

A Brave First Step

Much of this book is written specifically for mothers and some of it is intended for fathers and partners also, but the practice of mindfulness is one that will greatly benefit both parents in pregnancy, childbirth and parenthood. This book is offered as a nurturing guide to using mindfulness skills in developing more awareness, presence, compassion and well-being in your remarkable parenting journeys together. By reading these pages you are taking a brave first step, and if you can just be consciously present now, in this moment, with an open heart, you will be in a great starting place.

Many blessings on your way!

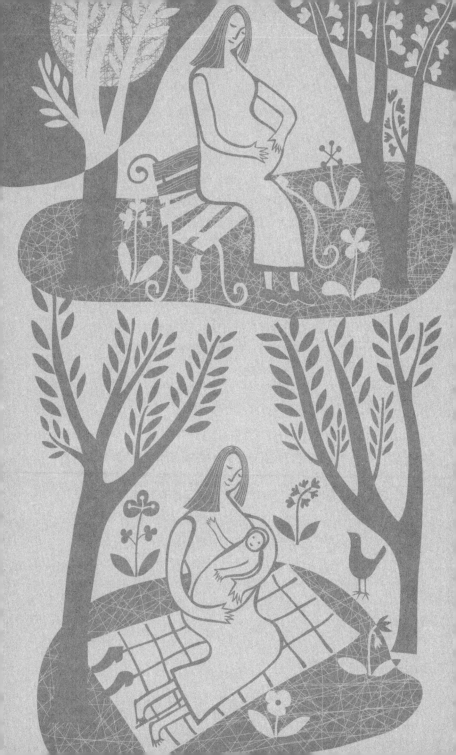

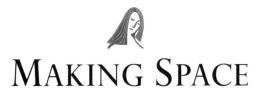

CHAPTER ONE

MAKING SPACE

When we speak of making something, it
usually entails creating, manipulating, forming
or conducting of some kind. In pregnancy, our bodies
are wrapped up in doing all of these things on a grand
scale. But in the act of making space in ourselves
through mindfulness, none of these things apply.
Here we can engage in an act of not doing, of not
changing, but simply of 'being' in our experience.
And as we do so, we may remember that life
is not just about doing.

A New Life Dawns Within Us

◆

As our body makes space in our womb for new life, so our heart and mind can also open up to the possibility of creating a new focus of awareness, from moment to moment.

WHEN WE ARRIVE at the time for conception and pregnancy in our lives, we bring with us our entire life stories so far. It's impossible not to. We are a collage of our journeys, our past experiences and the beliefs that have been forged in us along the way. Or at least it seems that way.

Yet with pregnancy we allow something new and very different to be created within us … a tiny life, whose newness borders on the revolutionary. A baby who we will learn to study, to sensitively discover and understand as they unravel so miraculously into being. And we have this unique period of growth that leads up to the first instant of our meeting.

Pregnancy is a phase in which to reconcile what has been with what will become. It is a process and a time of change, and even more so for a first-time mother. It is a recognition of our dreams for the future being in transit, in gestation, in the making. And all this is ongoing inside our bodies. At times, we can almost feel those cells multiplying and see our bellies enlarge. Then there are the flutterings of movement, the little feet stretching up under a rib or two. There is a lot going on in the womb, an entire human life in the making.

A Place of Listening

So what happens when we allow ourselves to become very quiet and to meet pregnancy in this moment, from a place of listening? The past and future recede in place of the present. Our preoccupations are diluted by breath, incoming and outgoing, rising and falling. Here we are able to recognize the 'is-ness' that exists everywhere and to notice our intrinsic connection with it. We may feel more expansive.

Life can get very spacious in this quiet place, when we are able to slow down and feel the vibrant effect that relaxation has on our entire being. Our muscles soften, our breathing eases, and gradually we begin to observe our thoughts without diving into them. This is an optimal experience in pregnancy, helping us to release the stresses of everyday life, as well as increasing our capacity to relax later on during childbirth and motherhood.

Pregnancy is a recognition of our dreams for the future being in transit

Through becoming more present-in-mind when we are pregnant, we bring our awareness into alignment with our bodies (and our babies), which exist and evolve physically in real time, right now. I see it as a way of making space in the continuing saga of our life stories. Essential space that will not only nourish us but will also help us to clear a pathway for the new life coming through us. A life we have already begun to care for though they are still so much a part of our own body.

The Busyness of Our Mind

Just imagine yourself as a room that is full of furniture, relics and artefacts from your unique life journey, and within these given parameters you need to arrange a spot for the cradle. 'Hmm,' you might say, 'what needs to go so I can fit my baby in here?' I think the only way to find the answer to this question is through the practice of space-making itself.

But often when we start to make space in our lives through meditation, we are faced head-on with the busyness of our mind. This can seem like white noise or a torrent of 'stuff' in the way of actually just sitting quietly. Thoughts and feelings that could have previously existed in our peripheral view might be revealed more fully. We may feel more confronted by all of this inner activity than if we were just going about our daily business, un-mindfully.

If doubt takes hold, we might begin to think 'Why am I doing this? I am sitting here being swamped with anything that my mind feels like churning up', and this can be disconcerting. Then come the questions of whether I'm doing this right, or whether I'm terrible at meditating, or whether this discipline should be left to those who have an innate disposition to inner peace. In fact, we could quite swiftly convince ourselves that we are just not cut out for the job.

Acceptance helps us to meet life as it is,
to meet ourselves as we are

ACCEPTANCE

◆

Finding a place of acceptance in ourselves can be both challenging and liberating. But as we begin to see that mindfulness practice is underpinned with acceptance, the whole process starts to make sense and the real inner work can be felt.

IN ALL OF THIS, IT IS ESSENTIAL TO REMEMBER that the core tenet of meditation is *acceptance*. This doesn't mean that to meditate we have to accept everything in our lives as it is. It doesn't mean being passive or living life in mediocrity. Our long-term intention for practising meditation might be to integrate a quality of openness and acceptance into the day-to-day. But of course we are human and we also need to create boundaries, to be assertive and to make judgements.

What it does mean is that when we enter into meditation, we do so with the understanding that everything about us and our experience can be met with acceptance. This gives us a navigation tool against the urge to control, change or

◆

The more clearly you understand
yourself and your emotions,
the more you become a lover of what is.

BARUCH SPINOZA (1632-1677)
EUROPEAN PHILOSOPHER

◆

♦

Mindfulness is the aware, balanced
acceptance of the present experience. It isn't more
complicated than that. It is opening to or receiving the
present moment, pleasant or unpleasant, just as it is,
without either clinging to it or rejecting it.

SYLVIA BOORSTEIN
AUTHOR, PSYCHOTHERAPIST, MEDITATION INSTRUCTOR

♦

---

judge what arises for us, because these will only suppress or manipulate our actual experience, which leads to an internal state of tension and conflict.

Acceptance helps us to meet life as it is, to meet ourselves as we are, and to 'be' with both of these in such a way that we do not create more resistance to them. We can even welcome and accept any resistance we may have to accepting, because from this place, we have the opportunity to perceive these momentary states of being with open awareness. When we accept the busyness, the spaciousness, the judgements or the sensations our bodies are enveloped by, we can be present with them, which may even change the way we experience them.

However, in the modern world we are not taught to value self-acceptance. We are conditioned to accept leaders, teachers and rules, but at a social and personal level we are given ideals to aim for and we are taught to continually better ourselves, based on stylized images of how we 'should' be.

So coming from this ingrained background of trying to achieve, to attain and to fit the model our culture deems desirable, the very notion of embracing acceptance in any practice might seem alien to us. But this is one of the reasons why mindfulness is so powerful in these times we live in, especially if we can approach acceptance not as something to achieve, but as an inherent part of ourselves that grows and matures in us, given the right inner environment.

Perfectly Imperfect

I believe that cultivating acceptance is especially beneficial for mothers, and women who are becoming mothers, because it can help us to be more authentic and to free ourselves of the desire to be perfect as we carry, birth and raise our little ones. For parents generally, at a very basic level it can support us to find our flow with life in each moment rather than struggling against it, and in this sense it is very empowering.

Step by step, we can work with acceptance in our lives, allowing it to inform our psyche and let it nourish our approach to raising children, without expectations of perfection from them either. We hold a lot of sway as parents and our influence makes an indelible mark on our children's life experience. This is a great responsibility and yet, by finding acceptance for our perfectly imperfect selves, we create more wellness within us, which enables us to naturally shine more vitality into their lives.

MINDFULNESS EXERCISE

ACCEPTANCE EXERCISE

Find a quiet time and place to do this exercise, when (hopefully) you won't be interrupted for about 10–15 minutes.

Make sure you are well supported if you are sitting or reclining. When you are ready, close or lower your eyes, whichever works better for you, and bring your attention to your breath as it enters and leaves your nose or mouth.

- Become aware of the sensations in your body as you inhale down into your chest and belly, and as you exhale.

- Remain awake to your breathing and when you find your focus drifting away, see if you can accept this and return your attention to your breath.

- As you continue to focus on your breath awareness, see if you can begin to bring this quality of acceptance into each and every aspect of your meditation experience.

- If you notice any tension or discomfort in your body, try again to meet it with acceptance. You can still change your position to get more comfortable if you need to.

- When thoughts, emotions, memories, future projections, hopes and fears emerge into your mind, just welcome them as they are, and return to your breath awareness.

Complete this exercise when you are ready and perhaps take a moment to reflect on it. You may want to make some notes in your journal. As the weeks go by, see how your relationship with acceptance develops.

Journaling

Keeping a journal can be a very useful tool for recording our observations and insights, and writing things down can also help us to stay alert to looping thoughts and emotional habits that keep us from living more in the present. It can be a way of getting things out, seeing them as they are and being less preoccupied by them, if at all.

If we are truly able to listen to the stirrings within, we gradually start to become more conscious of our 'stories' and see our patterns more objectively. We may at some point be able to identify and get some perspective on the inner routine of 'me', my beliefs, my habitual thoughts and feelings, which gives us a greater capacity to simply watch these playing out, without being drawn into them.

When we can recognize both conscious and unconscious threads interweaving and running through our lives, it is easier to see and track these as we meditate. Like a bird-watcher who has the identification book by her side and can say 'Hey, I know that hawk!'

I have written a series of questions, shown on the following page, which are intended to help you consciously explore what may be occupying most of your attention in daily life. This exercise is just an opportunity for you to journey a bit deeper into the most present themes in your life right now. Write as much as you wish, freely and without inhibition or self-judgement, and see what emerges.

MINDFUL EXERCISE

EXPLORING CURRENT THOUGHTS

- Take a few quiet moments for yourself and get comfortable, either sitting or lying down, with a pen and your journal to hand.
- Close or lower your eyes and just become aware of your breath.
- Notice the weight and contact of your body with where you are sitting or lying.
- Relax into your posture and focus your attention on your breath if you can. When it wanders, just gently return to this focus.
- When you are ready, ask yourself the following questions, trying to remain aware but not to judge any responses you have:

  What are my most common thoughts from day to day?

  What are my most common feelings from day to day?

  What do I hope for?

  What am I afraid of or worried by?

  What do I need?

  What, if anything, do I feel may be blocking me?

  What are other people's expectations of me and how do I feel about these?

  How do I feel about bringing a new life into this world?

  How do I feel about giving birth?

Be gentle with yourself as you reflect on your answers, because questions like these can touch on our vulnerabilities. Give yourself some time to digest them. You may have more questions to ask yourself after finishing this exercise and what you have written here may just feel like the tip of the iceberg in your personal explorations. Perhaps answers came up that you weren't expecting, opening new doors to your understanding.

PREPARING FOR MOTHERHOOD

◆

Pregnancy gives women a good opportunity to have quiet time and to gain insight or awareness into themselves. Making space for yourself in the midst of the whirlwind of life can hugely support your transition into motherhood, or into motherhood again.

T O ILLUSTRATE THE VALUE OF SPACE-MAKING, let me share with you some of my story and my first arrival into pregnancy. I was fortunate enough to have come across the practice of meditation at a young age and, even as a child, I was sometimes guided through visualizations or encouraged to find stillness while being in nature. I practised meditative exercises in my teens, and in my twenties took the leap into a more focused approach with the Buddhist Vipassana practice.

Vipassana means insight. It can also be likened to 'clear sight' or 'seeing deeply' into the true nature of reality. As a lead into practising Vipassana meditation, we start by becoming mindful of our breath and our physical sensations. When we are more aware of these, we can begin to watch our thoughts and emotions as they emerge and fade away from our inner-scape.

The purpose of this is not to disengage from who we are, but to begin to see ourselves as receivers and transmitters of information that does not define us, but which passes through, like lights and shadows that fleetingly touch the face of our true nature, which is infinite and deeply peaceful.

Finding Vipassana meditation was both difficult and freeing for me. I now had an incisive tool to help me reconnect with my inner still-point, from where everything became clearer and my 'being' was more centred in compassion – however, it was really hard work to have to confront my busy mind and find the patience I needed to watch it!

I came up with ways to avoid regular practice but would then go on retreats to immerse myself into the stillness once again, and slowly things began to shift. I gave up smoking and drinking. I gave up an unhelpful relationship and moved from the big city to a lively seaside town. And I began to see things in my life more clearly, knowing I had a place of refuge, sitting on that cushion and getting quiet enough to witness the noisy riot outpouring through my thinking mind.

A Meeting with Destiny

Strangely enough, it was in the midst of all of this change that I went on a retreat and bumped into the man who would later become the beloved father of my children. We can't have been paying too much attention to our breath, can we? But luckily, destiny was insistent that our paths should cross and if it happened to be on a meditation retreat, then so be it.

So just as my new life began to wind out of my old one, my new lover settled into it and with him came a deepening of my commitment to meditating. Nevertheless, it took us a full five years to be ready in ourselves for the journey into parenthood. It felt like a great unknown and we were slightly daunted by the prospect of such huge responsibility, though in truth I know I was deeply longing for a child.

Coming from a 'broken home' myself, I was also concerned that my children would not have to suffer the dysfunctional dynamics that can play out in families. In fact, I was fearful of this, which led me to develop super-human expectations of myself and my husband, and of our partnership.

Smoothing Out the Creases

So, as part of my preparation for *super-motherhood* during pregnancy, I decided to work with an Integrative Arts Psychotherapist to help smooth out some of the creases in my life, to understand my feelings and reactions better and to feel more supported. This proved an invaluable choice and it gave me a regular slot every week to talk and uncover my inner world.

During these sessions I sometimes painted, but perhaps because I already had a meditation practice, my preferred mode of self-exploration was through discussion and sitting with eyes closed, just noticing what arose within me. It began a little like watching the mind, but was different in that we went on to focus on specific feelings, which gave rise to sequences of inner images that were new every time. By bringing my conscious awareness to this film-like reflection unfolding inside me, and with gentle guidance, I was able to find meaning and insight into my unconscious mind.

I arrived into my pregnancy with issues and insecurities stemming from a complex childhood, but in making the space to connect with my unconscious self, I began to feel that *I* was actually the one with the answers to my own questions.

This was very empowering and I am so grateful for the opportunity to do this, as I know it greatly oiled the wheels of that smooth first pregnancy. I embraced my changing body. I adored the small being growing inside me and sang and spoke to it a lot. I felt womanly and grounded. There were moments of vulnerability too, but I knew I was resourced enough to find strength in my inner sense of connection.

Deepening my self-awareness definitely helped me through pregnancy, which may have otherwise been an emotional rollercoaster ride. And having worked with pregnant women for many years since, I know my experience was not unique.

A Hothouse of Hormones

Emotional issues can become more significant for women during the perinatal year. A woman becomes like a living hothouse of hormones in order to make, birth and feed a baby and she will potentially feel the psychological or emotional effects of this, just as plainly as her body will urge her to crave any nutrients it needs to supply its baby-making demands. In some ways, our bodies' chemistry just takes over.

Pregnancy also comes in phases. We may feel nauseous and delicate for a time and then perhaps blooming, radiant and invincible. We might experience emotion without necessarily understanding why and it can be challenging to ride the waves of our hormonally charged feelings in a world that avoids expressing strong emotions. It can trigger a sense of shame or embarrassment, yet it is completely normal and natural.

There are also specific areas of our lives that might be highlighted or placed under pressure during pregnancy, such as our immediate familial environment, our closest partnership, our existing children, health, work and finances. The state of play in all of these will influence how we feel, and cultivating our awareness can prove helpful in dealing with these.

BECOMING LIKE THE EYE OF THE STORM

I am here and the world revolves around me, while another world revolves within me. This process of creating a new life can bring inner turbulence, inner joy and many distinct waves of emotion. So if I am the meeting place between these worlds, where is my centre?

IT IS IMPORTANT NOT TO DISMISS our emotional world, as it is usually pointing us towards what needs our loving attention. Too often, people discredit and devalue their own feelings with judgements that crush their significance. But consider this situation as if, metaphorically, your sewer is blocked (a personal pattern or issue is triggered) and a repair person arrives at your house (in the form of your emotions) and you close the door saying, 'No thanks, it's really nothing.' If you ignore those feelings, you are going to be very sorry when your bowels need to move!

Emotions are our indicators of what is out of balance, what we can look at or change our relationship with and what we might want to leave behind us. Physiologically, the effect of crying helps us to release stress and to relax, and if we can see our emotions in this light, as messengers and catalysts, and give them the space to make themselves known to us, they are extremely valuable.

However, experiencing feelings can also be painful. So much so that we might prefer to just switch on the TV, check our phones, eat chocolate or engage with just about anything that distracts us from having to confront them.

Welcome Everything

What, then, is needed for us to be able to meet our feelings as they are, even when we are reacting with this fear of pain? When we approach emotions using mindfulness, the practice we follow is to be present with our experience and to meet it with a quality of enquiry and openness. That includes the fear and the pain. Everything – emotion, thought, yearning, resistance, everything in our experience has permission to be present. And we watch it unfold before us. It sounds simple, but that doesn't mean it's easy. It is a practice and it takes time to find our way with it.

We don't like how difficult emotions feel …

We don't know what to do with the discomfort

and vulnerability. Emotion can feel terrible, even

physically overwhelming. We can feel exposed,

at risk and uncertain in the midst of emotion.

Our instinct is to run from pain.

FROM 'RISING STRONG'
BRENÉ BROWN

When we develop a regular meditation practice over time, we become more present to our feelings and it becomes easier to hold our emotional life with compassion. It is not that we get 'better' at doing this, but in a way we get more used to it, and perhaps more dedicated. However, becoming present to difficult emotions in ourselves can be really hard. Have you ever tried to become more mindful when you are in a rage? Or experiencing grief? It is not easy at all.

The Witness

In the following exercise, I invite you to connect with your emotions and, as you do so, try to bring to them your non-judgemental awareness. While doing this, you may notice that they change. They might become less all-encompassing or just hold less of a charge for you. And they might not. Try to be open to whatever you perceive.

But the key to mindfulness is to know that, whatever emotional state we are in, no matter how wild or vulnerable, there is also a part of us inside that just witnesses. And the more we get to know this part, the more we begin to recognize that although it is very quiet, our inner witness is always present. You may even realize that this witness aspect of you is there in your dreams. It just watches, as if your dream or your life or your mind is a movie.

It is also at the heart of meditation practice and in some ways the very act of meditating is simply one of choosing to be with the witness, rather than with the 'story' side of the mind. When we identify less with the stories that charge through us, with this drama and that, and instead focus on watching them with our full awareness, we gradually give our consciousness permission to change.

It is not that we lose interest or stop caring about things that may be very real for us. It is not that we disengage. Being with the witness gives us an opportunity to rest in the present moment and to be with whatever that brings. When we are assailed by thoughts, as we will be in meditation, watching this mental busyness from a place of witnessing, rather than participating in it, is one way home to awareness. It is our chance to become present, which is a nourishing experience. Being with the witness also airs and opens up the narrow scope of our busy thinking minds, making us available to greater insight, understanding and compassion.

MINDFUL EXERCISE

CONNECTING WITH YOUR INNER WITNESS

The following exercise can be done at any time, but see if it is also possible for you to practise it when you are immersed in any strong or difficult emotions.

- Find a quiet space to sit and get into a comfortable position.
- Close or lower your eyes and start to become aware of your breath as it enters and leaves your nose or mouth.
- Notice each inhalation dropping down into your body and each exhalation leaving your body through your nose or mouth. If your mind wanders, just come back to your breath.
- Observe any physical sensations in your body and when your attention drifts, return it to your sensations and to your breath.
- Now bring to mind an issue in your life that may generate tricky or challenging emotions for you and notice how you feel.
- What physical sensations arise in the presence of this emotion?
- Just be with these feelings and sensations in the present moment, and for now, try to let go of the 'story' attached to the issue, with its past and future implications.
- Bring your full conscious awareness to your emotions and body.
- Let your breath continue to anchor your attention into this moment and just witness the feelings you are experiencing.
- Keep witnessing, and if judgements about your feelings appear, simply witness those thoughts too.
- When you are ready to complete this exercise, open your eyes fully and give yourself time to reflect on and take note of anything you discovered about your experience.

Simply Be with Your Feelings

There is no censorship of feelings in this work, just a turning to face them. The witness has no judgement of what it sees, it just sees. When we meet strong emotions with our complete presence, it can release the intensity of our experience, or increase it. Neither of these outcomes, however, is the aim of meditation. By meditating, we are just trying to be with those feelings without changing them at all. We can observe how we feel them, and follow how they fluctuate and change, but we don't need to control them. And if we notice a part of ourselves wanting to control or change our experience, we can also observe this part, with acceptance.

The Witness & the Thinker

Becoming familiar with your inner witness brings to light a new relationship with two aspects of yourself: the one who is *in* thought and the one who *watches* the thought. We may continually fluctuate between these two viewpoints as we sit in meditation, and this is fine – in fact, we need the thinker part of ourselves to even begin to know the witness and vice versa.

The 'thinker' is an important part of being human, enabling us to plan and reflect, to calculate, analyse and engage with the world as an identified being, ego or self, which we *are* in physical form. However, in human life, and especially in the lives we lead today, the thinker can dominate our potential to live in an expansive experience of the present.

The witness allows us to step out of our craving to control, to escape or to blame. It offers us a sanctuary from being identified with the self through noticing our thoughts and feelings instead, as part of the phenomenon of life, arising and fading away. We still think and feel, yet with the witness side of ourselves activated, we are able to anchor our experiences in conscious awareness. By engaging with the witness, we can be with our 'thinker' more mindfully.

PHYSICAL DISCOMFORT IN PREGNANCY

◆

What we experience physically during pregnancy and birth is not comparable to any other physical experience. We embark on a journey that spans a spectrum of physical states, needs and responses, at times requiring a level of surrender previously unimaginable to us.

IN PREGNANCY, THERE MAY BE INSTANCES when we feel sick as dogs; others when we feel heavy, exhausted and immobile. Sometimes we may crave orange juice, spinach, meat, milk or cake with wild abandon, at three in the morning. Sometimes we might feel ourselves to be the embodiment of vitality and at other times sleep is our only goal.

And there will be moments when we get sore. Although many of us have comfortable pregnancies, it is not uncommon for women to have physical discomfort for much of this gestational phase, which can be very difficult to deal with.

Experiencing even temporary discomfort can floor us. And pain is a theme that can show up at any time throughout the whole perinatal year as we transition from pregnancy to labour to birth, to post-birth and breastfeeding.

So how can we work mindfully with these physical challenges, and will it help us? Well, I have never personally experienced mindfulness as a 'cure' for pain; however, it has given me another way of responding to it. Our natural reaction to pain is one of aversion. We resist it. Intense pain immediately sends signals to the brain that we are in danger, which wakes us up to a potential life threat.

Mindfulness practice gives us another way of responding to pain

While low-level discomfort can bring up emotions such as sadness, irritation and anxiety, with mindfulness practice we can become aware of our physical sensations and witness our response to them. If we notice the mind creating a story about how bad they are or how we wish they would go away, we can become aware of this and find acceptance for our story too.

Listen to the Pain

If you are experiencing physical discomfort, try using the Inner Witness exercise to help you to *be* with it. Sometimes, by giving our complete attention and acceptance to an aching or soreness, it changes, or sometimes our feelings and judgements about it can change. Even the practice of focusing on our breath during an experience of pain can help to keep the mind clear and relax the body so that sensations naturally reduce in intensity. Just be aware of what you find, though, without trying to premeditate or create an outcome. And also listen to your intuition and common sense – if you feel that this pain is present for a reason and you want a professional opinion, follow your hunch and seek advice.

We will continue to focus on physical sensations throughout this book. But mindfully exploring any discomfort in pregnancy is actually excellent practice for the possibility of being with intense sensations during labour and birth, so if you can see this as an opportunity, it could be very helpful.

COMPASSION

◆

When we make space inside ourselves through cultivating awareness, the heart will open, in its own time. We may not notice this to begin with, but it will open up eventually and when it does, meditation becomes an experience of kindness. This, in all its simplicity, is a spiritual experience.

COMPASSION LIES BEHIND THE PRACTICE of meeting our experience with acceptance. It is not always obvious and it may not be recognizable in the form of a 'loving' feeling. It may be encountered as a sense of peace, or we may find ourselves spontaneously responding to something in our thoughts with kindness rather than judgement. When we integrate mindfulness into our lives, we might notice a shift in our general outlook from one of criticism or blame, either of self or others, to one of trying to understand or to benefit all.

But the further we venture into meditation, the clearer it becomes that we have a shared experience, connection and investment with all life. Understanding this might change our vision from a conditioned, polarized sense of 'us and them' to simply understanding there is 'us'. And as we are sitting with 'what is' in meditation, an intelligence or awakening can naturally manifest in us, tuning us in to this universal truth. We don't have to think about it, convince ourselves or anticipate it to be able to 'know' this, but we may begin to consciously understand it through experience.

Parenting & Unity

Understanding that we are part of something greater than ourselves can also be experienced in pregnancy, childbirth, and through becoming a mother. For example, you may notice a feeling of camaraderie, a sense of sisterhood with other pregnant women, regardless of differences in age, race or background. Our common experience provides a pathway of 'knowing' that crosses the borders of language and culture.

I find this a beautiful aspect of the motherhood journey and I remember, when I was first pregnant, the feeling of almost joining a 'club' with all mothers. Parenthood is an initiation, particularly for women, who physically gestate their babies and cross the threshold of birth. The sense of connection with this universal tribe of mothers can intensify during childbirth, when a mother's intuition is heightened, and many mothers do experience the feeling that they are labouring alongside all the women giving birth around the world at the same time. We can feel supported by this, knowing that we are not alone.

In fact, it is just this quality of sisterhood that has ensured our survival and development as a human species on Earth. Women, young and old, have always gathered together at every stage of life, to share. For millennia, we have shared child rearing, breastfed each other's babies, taught each other skills for birth, celebrated newborns, honoured our girls' menarches and learned from women experiencing menopause and from wise elders. Without this female support and 'holding', our ancestors would not have flourished into the thriving populations we have on this planet today.

In developing compassion, perhaps one
could begin with the wish that oneself be free of
suffering, and then take that natural feeling towards
oneself and cultivate it, enhance it and extend it
out to include and embrace others.

THE DALAI LAMA
TIBETAN SPIRITUAL LEADER AND TEACHER

Beyond Self

Our ability to tap into the feeling of commonality as mothers supports us to do what we do, which is a lot. I remember many situations as a new mother where I would be holding or carrying my baby and would meet another woman, a stranger, cradling her own newborn, and I could not help but feel empathy and interest, both for her and her child. Or at times when a friend or neighbour had just given birth, noticing my instinctive urge to offer help, even if I already had a lot of maternal responsibilities myself. And fathers can feel the same sense of brotherhood in this way. Compassion and empathy play a big role in parenting.

So if bringing a new life into the world naturally increases our ability to experience our human connection and compassion, how do we enable this feeling of compassion to support our practice of mindfulness? To explore this, we first need to locate the meeting point between compassion and developing a wider sense of responsibility.

Compassion is like a mature form of empathy that sees beyond judgement. It can be experienced as a feeling or attitude that is non-grasping, non-dualistic, but imbued with acceptance. But there is something more: compassion involves a willingness to help and benefit all of life.

Compassion and empathy
play a big role in parenting

The experience of compassion takes mindfulness practice to another level; our experience becomes more spacious and connected. This quality of loving-kindness also helps to free us from the human but small-minded need to control, or from egoic clinging to 'me', 'my identity', 'my life'. Instead, it brings the insight that all beings feel. And so whatever arises in our meditation can be met with a deeper sense of our common, sentient unity. But it must begin with compassion for ourselves, as we are the spring-source from which it can flow outwards towards others.

Loving-Kindness

There is a powerful teaching attributed to the Buddha, called the Metta Sutta, or Unlimited Kindness Sutra, which has been applied in Buddhism as a practice called Metta Bhavana, its closest translation being 'loving-kindness meditation'. It calls on practitioners to generate a feeling of compassion, initially for themselves, then for others, and ultimately for everything that lives. As an inner process, it can actually change our approach to life if it is practised regularly, and if everyone practised it, on a regular basis, this would undoubtedly change the world. But you do not need to be a Buddhist to feel the value of practising Metta because, as we have seen, loving-kindness is a feeling that is common to us all. And this practice is very much about recognising that deep down we all share the need for it.

MINDFUL EXERCISE

METTA BHAVANA

Please don't rush through this practice — give yourself time between each step to pause and connect with your feelings of compassion. Find a comfortable sitting position and allow the mind to settle by beginning to focus on your breath.

- Take a moment to reflect on yourself; consider all that you do in your life to benefit yourself and others. Spend some time generating compassion for yourself in all your human-ness, for the challenges you may have experienced and for your innate wish for health and happiness. You can include your baby in this and cultivate love for both of you.

- Now bring to mind someone you love (but not a partner) and begin to send the same quality of compassion to them, reflecting on all that they do in their lives to benefit themselves and others. Consider the challenges they may have experienced, their human-ness and their inner wish for well-being and happiness too.

- Next bring to mind someone who brings up difficult thoughts or feelings for you. Reflect for a moment on all that they do in their lives to try to benefit themselves and others. Consider the challenges they may also have faced in their life, their human-ness and their own deeper wish to be well and happy. Try to generate the same quality of kindness and compassion for this person.

- Then bring to mind a stranger, someone you may have seen or met a few times but hardly know, and try to cultivate a feeling of care and empathy for this person. Reflect on their efforts to benefit themselves and others. Consider their human-ness, that they too may have experienced challenges in their life and that they also wish for health and happiness.
- Now visualize your closer community, people you know and interact with from day to day; see them as a group of people and send out feelings of kindness to them. Consider the human challenges that these people may face and the efforts made by everyone here to benefit themselves and others and to lead happy lives.
- Now imagine this feeling of compassion spreading further outward into other communities and, gradually, throughout the entire country in which you live. And continue to visualize this feeling expanding into other countries and communities, bringing this quality of loving-kindness to all beings, human, animal, bird, fish, insect, plant, etc, so that eventually you imagine the whole world enveloped in this feeling of compassion.
- Then send compassion out into the universe and to all life beyond this world.

When you have completed this meditation, try to make some time to write about your experience of it, especially if it is the first time you have tried doing the Metta Bhavana practice, because its impact can be very significant.

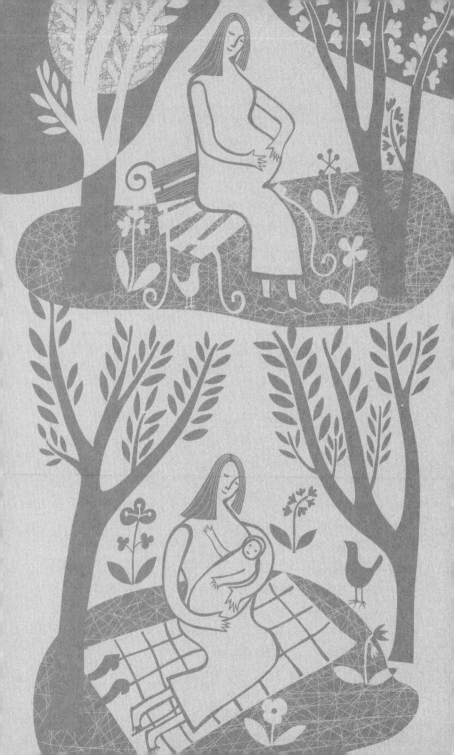

CHAPTER TWO

THE PREGNANT PAUSE

When we slow down, we can begin to listen.
When we listen, we can start to hear, and in hearing
with an open mind, we can let go of whatever we were
holding on to and be present in this moment. By gently
pressing the pause button on our busy itineraries from
time to time, each day, we can generously offer
ourselves the chance to be here and now. And when
we consider the busy phase of parenting a newborn
that lies ahead of us, this becomes an essential
prerequisite to it all.

Awakening

◆

To be awake, to be consciously present, is simply to allow all of our experience in. We can welcome this sense of being by opening our hearts, our minds, our senses and perceptions to full capacity. This magic is heightened in pregnancy, as we experience two lives in one.

I HAVE ONLY BEEN PREGNANT TWICE and am the grateful mother of two children. Pregnancy was a fascinating time for me on both occasions, a time of keenly observing my changing physiology, my thinking-feeling world, and the mysterious new being growing inside me. During my second pregnancy, though, I wished my life could have been quieter as I already had a small child to care for and my body wanted more time to rest.

Unfortunately, this didn't happen, and I ended up with a stubborn and painful chest infection. During the time that followed, leading up to my son's birth, I would take myself off in the evenings and meditate as often as I could. It was as though there was something I needed that I could only find in this quiet time alone. I remember the relief I felt, sitting cross-legged on my pillows, finally able to receive the nourishment I had been yearning for all day. The simplicity of sitting and breathing was like an elixir for my busy tiredness.

On reflection it's surprising that I was able to sit in awareness for much of the time without falling asleep, but often I did, and it became my soul food. Taking the opportunity to stop in this way was exactly what I needed and I believe that this is a natural necessity in pregnancy. Yet we live in a world that requires us to keep going, even when we are tired. We are expected to take a hit of caffeine or sugar to raise our energy levels and to meet the demands of modern life when our bodies are telling us otherwise.

Retreating in Pregnancy

In pregnancy, our inner environment, visible only because of our bellies and perhaps slightly swollen limbs, is very different. In chemistry, in physical organization, in body-fluid proportions, in the bearing of weight and the stretching of skin, we change dramatically. Internally, we are temporarily a different woman, nurturing a new human life; yet externally, in the way we live, it's business as usual.

Some tribal cultures around the world have traditionally held women's physiological processes in high regard as sacred rites. Menstruation, among certain Native American tribal people such as the Lakota, is revered as a personal ceremonial event in a woman's life each month. During her 'moon-time', or period, a Lakota woman was traditionally given space from her participation in community work, to be in prayer on behalf of herself and her people. To see the spiritual power unique to a woman's physiology shows a people who can listen deeply to nature. In Westernized culture, however,

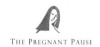
menstruation is practically taboo and menopause is seldom discussed in public, while birth is mainly considered to be an unsafe medical event that should happen in hospitals, where it can be controlled.

But I believe that if we lived in a world that had been shaped by women and men in balance with each other and with our natural environment, we would be honouring these essential phases in a woman's life, such as menstruation, pregnancy and birth, as times in which rest and space are required.

Pregnancy in Modern Times

In her book *Welcoming Spirit Home*, Sobonfu Somé, spiritual teacher from the Dagara tribe in Burkina Faso, writes about conception and pregnancy as significant phases in which both mother and father engage in ceremonies to prepare themselves to receive their child. During pregnancy, parents undertake specific inner work and self-healing for the important role of nurturing the spirit who will come through them.

I feel it is so important to look at our modern attitudes to pregnancy and birth in contrast to those of older cultures. As we find the vast distinctions between them, it helps us gain some perspective on our contemporary outlook, which we take for granted as the norm. And once we can see this clearly, it can help us to see through it. Pregnancy and birth are not merely a mechanical kind of bodily process that result in a baby. They are so much more than this, and so are we.

Today, Scandinavian countries such as Sweden and Norway have put in place some exceptional parental rights, including extended paid leave that can be shared between parents when their baby is born. In doing this, they have instilled a cultural value for mothers, babies, fathers and partners. They have publicly prized the health of 'the family' itself above the family's vocational productivity, and in doing so they also demonstrate due respect for the intense job of child-rearing, which both parents can contribute to.

Honouring Pregnancy

This is unusual for modern countries, and as we emerge from the past several millennia, in which a predominantly male society has been constructed and adhered to, we can see that women's subjects are not high profile. Many women continue to work right through pregnancy and into their third trimester, leaving little time to hunker down and relax before birth.

But pregnancy and birth have not always been like this and they do not have to be like this. We *can* bring more choice into our lives and we *can* create resting places in the busy flood of daily activity to make this time more relaxed. My sense is that we need to remember how to live at a different pace. As human beings, we have all grown in the womb ourselves and have some kind of memory of what it is to be simply sentient. We all sleep, which involves relaxation, so we each hold the blueprint of how to relax deeply.

Make an Intention

We can make an intention to include in our waking hours interludes of physical and mental rest, even if they are just momentary, fleeting glimpses of our lives, in full awareness. And if we do, we will be giving ourselves the gift of honouring our pregnancies, regardless of what the rest of the world around us is doing.

When I was pregnant, on both occasions, I took time out to go on a yoga and meditation retreat. This felt very important for me, to have the space to give up my responsibilities for a while, to be guided, to rest and to be nourished on so many levels, including being cooked for! In fact, the retreat I attended during my second pregnancy was right at the end of my first trimester and over the course of those three days, every trace of the potent nausea I had been feeling was gone. So in the knowledge that mothers inspire each other, I hope you too can create the opportunity to make this happen in your pregnancy. This special time might bring you a window of rest that you didn't even realise you needed so much.

---◆---

Sitting peacefully, I smile

The new day begins,

I make a vow to live deeply, mindfully.

THICH NHAT HANH
VIETNAMESE BUDDHIST MONK AND PEACE ACTIVIST

---◆---

PRESSING THE PAUSE BUTTON

◆

Life slows down of its own accord when we start to make spaces for that to happen. As we live, so we create, and we can masterfully influence the direction and speed we travel in by choosing to rest, to listen and to watch for a moment, between moments.

As I WRITE THIS, IT IS AUTUMN and the view from my glass-walled office is of golden and rust-coloured leaves, some scattered on the ground and some still clinging to the twigs and branches of the surrounding trees. Since sitting here, it has dawned on me that each of these luminous leaves has grown and lived on their tree for many months and when one of them falls, this journey is the leaf's dance to the Earth. It happens only once.

Somehow this feels significant to me, like birth; it happens for a child only once. And it is also a dance, between mother and baby, a falling to Earth. When we notice the profound within the everyday, this can awaken our understanding that each moment is precious and new, just as when we understand the newness of each moment we can see its profundity. Here we meet with the notion of 'shoshin', or beginner's mind, in Zen Buddhism. Beginner's mind is the cultivation of an outlook on life that is always fresh and full of possibilities. This brings an aliveness to the way we approach our daily activities and our awareness of the world around us.

The Newness of Now

Shunryu Suzuki, the Japanese Zen monk who helped to popularize Zen Buddhism in the US, once said that as soon as we see something, we already begin to intellectualize it and as soon as we intellectualize it, it is no longer what we saw. This is so true of the way we usually go about things from day to day, functioning on schedule, in such a way that our lives are pre-conceived and planned before we have even lived them. We forget that this moment now is new, even

Life constantly renews, reinvents and births itself afresh

if we are involved in an activity we have done many times before. As we try to predetermine the acts we are engaged in, we forget that these are part of our ephemeral existence, which is relentlessly changing, emerging and fading out. It is so valuable to take this approach into life, recognizing that not only is this moment new, but that it will never happen again in the same way.

This car journey, this feeling of sunlight on skin, this constellation of clouds or people or leaves is unique and transient. Life doesn't repeat itself; it constantly changes, renews, reinvents and births itself afresh. And as we participate in this miraculous dance of moments, sometimes we fall asleep on our feet, and we lose our steps. Sometimes we forget them, but each of us holds the potential to remember and we can always reawaken when we choose to.

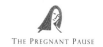

MINDFUL EXERCISE

WAKING TO THIS MOMENT

Try to take this exercise into your daily life and apply it to whatever
you are doing, even if that is only for a few seconds. You can use it
to wake up to the present experience you are having and see how
it affects this.

While you are engaged in any activity, try to remember to say to
yourself from time to time, 'I am here'.

- Initially, become aware of your breathing and watch its flow as
  you inhale and exhale.
- Then notice your facial expression and posture, sensing any tension or tightness you may be holding in your muscles.
- Then bring your attention to any other physical sensations in your
  body. These may be related to the action you are involved in,
  whether it is walking, sitting, standing, speaking, preparing or
  eating food, and so on.
- Notice any emotions or thoughts that are present right now.
- Then start to bring your awareness to your environment through
  your senses: vision, hearing, smell, taste and feeling, through the
  air around you, temperature, etc.
- Sustain your engagement with this practice for as long as possible
  each time you do it, but don't worry if that is only 30 seconds.

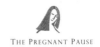

In time, as you practise Waking to this Moment, it will become a more integrated part of your general awareness, and this is a wonderful experience. As it becomes a way of life, it accompanies the realization that this is what it is to live. If you have ever felt before that you were being 'lived' or directed by your thoughts, then 'waking to this moment' enables you to step away from that entrapment and to begin to consciously receive the riches of life, as it is.

Absorbing Nature

Being in nature mindfully is the most wonderful time to relax. Japanese haiku verse, pioneered by poets such as Basho and Shiki right up to the modern day, has often been dedicated to meditations on the wonders of the natural world in its immense simplicity. This is just one example of the inspirational impact that nature continues to have upon us, but there are so many. And for millennia, we as a species have lived in nature's pocket, our lives completely enmeshed with her creations and cycles.

Early Autumn —

Rice field, ocean,

One green.

MATSUO BASHO 1644–94
JAPANESE POET

Today, many of us are less connected with the earth than we have ever been, and children are growing up with little knowledge of nature. Living in an urban terrain can make it more difficult to find nature-spaces, but there are opportunities to engage that we might sometimes overlook.

For example, we all live with the sky above us, in its ever-changing colours and garments of cloud wool and lace, its light-filled celestial bodies that shine through our atmosphere from night into day and day into night. And the drift of birds, insects, falling rain or snow can draw our attention to the wind and the quality of the air's movements. Taking time to look at the sky and feel the breeze or stillness, even on a grey day, can help us to become really present and to value the natural reservoir of air around us.

Reaching the Still Place

The closer we live to trees, gardens, parks, forests, coastlines, mountains, meadows, valleys and wild open spaces, the easier it is for us to take time to nestle into the beauty of our natural world. And if we really tune in and listen to our needs in pregnancy, I believe there is an innate calling in us to ground ourselves. There is a reason our ancestors in so many cultures saw the Earth as the Great Mother. She perpetually gives birth, and when we are in labour, it is our relationship to gravity and the earth that can assist the passage of our babies down and through us.

Connecting with the ground beneath us can slow us down. As we reach a still place in ourselves, we notice our physical points of contact with the earth, the sensations on the surface of our body where our skin meets the air. We let all our senses drink in the manifest world around us, its colours, shapes and textures; its smells and sounds, like a feast of perhaps ordinary yet remarkable phenomena.

And maybe most importantly of all, the enjoyment of being in nature during pregnancy combines two essential contributing factors to our body's production of oxytocin (our 'love' hormone, essential for labour and birth), which are relaxation and happiness. Nature's influence enables us to release stress and through it we can access a feeling of connection to something greater than ourselves, making it the most potent schoolroom for us to cultivate mindfulness practice.

◆

When your world moves too fast
and you lose yourself in the chaos,
introduce yourself to each colour of the sunset.
Reacquaint yourself with the Earth beneath your feet.
Thank the air that surrounds you
with every breath you take.
Find yourself in the appreciation of life.

CHRISTY ANN MARTINE
CANADIAN POET

◆

GETTING CURIOUS ABOUT YOUR PREGNANCY

◆

Are you listening? As we become quiet enough to listen and feel, we find the workings of our own body — the heartbeat, the pulse, the sound of our digestion. This is the world in which a baby swims, grows, sleeps and is wakeful. Can you feel your baby?

THE WORK I DO WITH PREGNANT MOTHERS always supports them to build a sense of connection with the unborn child they are carrying. Communicating with our babes in utero can involve speech, sound and song, or movement, touch and physical vibration. During both of my pregnancies, I also used to simply place my hands on my belly and send them my love, and I sensed that they got it. This practice of communicating with your baby in utero has now been scientifically recognized as playing a role in their development beyond birth. And many mothers will recount stories of babies kicking or moving inside them to sequential bouts of stimulus like sounds or tapping on their bellies, etc. Songs we sing or music we play to our babies in utero can continue to produce a response of stimulation or calm, during their first few months of life especially.

Whether or not we are aware of it at the time, there are also things we perceive about our little ones before they are born, even if those things just seem instinctual to us. For example, my elder child has always disliked loud music and

MINDFUL EXERCISE

LISTENING TO YOUR BABY

This exercise can be done with both parents at any time, but it is especially good to do it at a time when the little one is moving around so that both can feel it.

It is helpful if you can sit or lie down during this exercise, and you can have your eyes open or closed. If both parents are present, find a position between you so that all four of your hands can rest comfortably on the belly.

- **Mothers:** relax your breathing and become aware of any physical sensations in your womb, especially your baby's movement.
- **Both parents:** keep 'listening' and, as you do so, soften in your own bodies and relax more deeply.
- Notice any physical vibrations of your baby's movements through your hands from the surface of the belly, too.
- Try to be with this experience without too much thinking, but just observing the sensations.
- Notice any emotions arising also.
- Cultivate some love for yourselves and your baby.

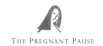
when she was in my womb I would feel the urge to run away from noisy speakers, while my younger one loves loud music and during my pregnancy with him, I'd be the one standing by the sound system at a dance.

So during our nine or so months together, we are learning about each other, through each other, which is a very special opportunity for bonding before birth. Mothers are inherently very connected to their babies in pregnancy, even unconsciously, but it is also lovely to tune in to them using the skills of mindfulness practice.

Flexing Limbs

Being pregnant is a temporal state. So many women I meet, especially when they are busy mothers already, tell me that their current pregnancy has 'flown past'. And it is really easy for that to happen when we are getting on with our lives. But making time to be really present when your child is moving around in the womb is one way of becoming more conscious in your experience of pregnancy, even if your awareness is only held there briefly.

I still have an enduring memory of sitting at home in my ninth month of pregnancy and feeling a little foot pressing into my ribs. The foot belonged to a long leg that I sensed was stretching up under my diaphragm and liver. The small being inside me was flexing her limbs and I recall thinking, is this okay? Will my body be able to accommodate my baby's yoga?

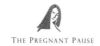
It felt strange, as if I needed to catch my breath, and I laughed at how bizarre it was to have another human being inside me, with their own agenda!

Only a pregnant woman can know this kind of experience – the feeling of kicking from inside the womb, the occasional scratching with little fingernails, the poking elbow or knee, and the bumping sensation of her baby's head against her cervix as she walks down the street in late pregnancy. It is extraordinary, and becomes more so as the birth gets closer.

PRELUDE TO BIRTH

In late pregnancy, as we prepare ourselves for the physiological transition of labour, birth and caring for our newborn child, many other aspects of our world, from the emotional, spiritual and practical to the way we think about life, will also be transformed and redefined.

As you approach the last few months of your pregnancy, keep noticing your feelings about the coming birth. Become aware of questions or thoughts that arise for you, and observe your intuitions, instinctual urges and dreams. The prospect of giving birth can bring both fear and excitement with it. Fear is especially important to recognize, as it can generate inner levels of tension and stress hormones, which are not compatible with the beneficial birth hormones, such as oxytocin, that naturally build up in us towards labour.

Sometimes, facing fears – speaking and naming them, writing them down and sharing them – helps to alleviate their hold on us. If you are experiencing fear about childbirth, even if it's just a faint concern, use some journal pages to write about it and get to know it without judging or trying to change it in any way. What is your fear about? Where do you think it comes from? What thoughts does it bring? When do you feel fearful? What do you think might diminish your fear?

The Inner Narrative

As you do this, you may notice whether the fear you have been holding feels out of proportion. It may also be possible to see if your fears or apprehensions about the impending birth are about crossing new or old territory. Fears based on past experiences or stories can run deep and hugely interfere with our ability to be open to the present; while fear of the unknown can be equally limiting, taking us out of this moment and into a projected, imagined future reality. And sometimes these past and future fears are linked together in one long timeline of fearful narrative.

A woman who is about to give birth may harbour a whole array of emotions about it, which is both normal and natural. However, in order to support herself emotionally, mentally and hormonally so that she feels at her best as she goes into labour, being unrestricted by fear is an optimal state. This is why practising mindfulness is so helpful in pregnancy, because

MINDFUL EXERCISE

BEING WITH FEAR

This exercise echoes the Inner Witness practice in chapter one, but we will focus specifically on getting to know fear, so it is helpful to practise it if you have been or are feeling fear or anxiety.

- Find a comfortable sitting or lying position and relax into your posture.
- Notice your breath as it flows into and out of your nose or mouth.
- Notice the rise and fall of your body as you breathe.
- Become aware of the weight and sensations of your body, and the pressure of your body against wherever you are sitting or lying.
- As you relax into this conscious presence, find where you are holding fear in your body.
- Notice the sensations of this fearful feeling.
- Begin naming the characteristics of these sensations, such as prickling, hot, aching, vibrating, piercing, cold, etc. You may even sense a colour to them.
- Hold these sensations in your present awareness.
- Now begin to notice any thoughts you have relating to this fear. Try not to get swept up in the thoughts themselves but just recognize and be conscious of them.
- See if you can bring a quality of acceptance to these feelings, sensations and thoughts, just allowing everything in your experience to be acceptable.
- If you are able to do this, you may notice a sense of compassion arising in yourself.
- If you can, just cultivate this feeling of kindness for yourself, and rest in this space for as long as you wish.

it can help us to build an inner space where we can be with emotions like fear without needing to change them, yet also without being governed by them.

Diminishing Fear

Fear is an emotion that all human beings feel. But when we can find acceptance, compassion and even relaxation in the face of it, its presence starts to lose power. This is because fear creates a tension in us – held within the body – and when the tension dissolves, the fear will also diminish. It is good to find some self-love at moments when we are triggered

Cultivate a feeling of kindness for yourself

into fear about something, in just the same way that we might feel love for someone else who is frightened. It is just so human, as are we, and when we care for the vulnerable parts of ourselves, we grow and deepen as people, and as parents.

Self-care is actually an essential part of preparing for birth and motherhood. And it can take many forms, from investing in a weekly massage to going to bed early, to stopping and resting every time we eat something. When we bear in mind that this is a special time to act on meeting our physical needs before the baby arrives, we can be more generous with ourselves than we would perhaps otherwise be. What may seem indulgent is actually just a way of tanking up before we embark on the next huge leg of the journey.

Love, the Flip Side of Fear

Self-care can also be about learning to love who we are and to overcome the areas where we lack self-acceptance. Motherhood is truly a path of love, and there are many aspects to this. These range from the physiological, where loving feelings actually hold the hormonal keys to birth and bonding, to the developmental, where our maternal instincts are able to evolve and flourish to their full potential when love is flowing in us. If we can focus on parenting with love, this will also have an impact on our wider families and communities, on the generation we are raising and on those who will follow. So having a precious inner resource of self-love is incredibly valuable for every step of our participation in this journey.

Love is like the flip side of fear and loving experiences have the capacity to melt stress and fearful reactions. Expressing it and receiving it can put us at ease with feelings of safety and happiness. But loving or accepting ourselves is not always easy. It takes commitment and practice and can require us to leap hurdles that might seem insurmountable, such as a lifetime of low self-worth, perhaps. In Metta Bhavana, self-compassion is pivotal to the deepening of compassion for others and this meditation can be a deeply nurturing practice, especially if you find self-love difficult. By cultivating love for ourselves, in the moments we remember, we begin to fill our own reservoir. This is not about narcissism, it is just a recognition of our human need for self-kindness.

Am I Worthy?

But we also have societal ideas about what love is and whether or not we deserve it and these can block our ability to feel love for ourselves. The mind gets in the way of the heart because many of us have been brought up in cultures that respect intellect and reason over authentic human feelings.

The quest to experience real self-compassion has been a theme running through my life for many years, because as a fully grown adult I have at times been beguiled by my own lack of it. There have been moments when I assumed that I was okay with who I am, only to turn a tricky bend and find I was pelting myself with mistrust, blame, shame and dislike. Although I have found a lot of personal healing along the way, there are still instances when this lack of love for myself prevails, and I need to return to my Metta practice. Because the purpose of loving-kindness meditation is to find the love within ourselves that is not performance-based. It is just love, as it is; like the core of love between a parent and child.

When you have pain within you, the first thing
to do is to bring the energy of mindfulness to embrace
the pain ... We must take care of our pain as
we would take care of our own baby.

FROM 'TRUE LOVE'
THICH NHAT HANH

Cultivating Self-love

If you are not used to this practice, it can take time to clarify this area around love and deserving, so I have written some questions to support your own explorations. You may find it useful to journal here, allowing your answers to flow without overthinking. My hope is that by responding to this exercise as honestly as you can, it will help you to deepen your Metta practice, so that it feels more authentic and real rather than just words or ideas.

- Am I deserving of love?
- Should I do something or be a certain way to be more deserving of love? (This can relate to your personal image, lifestyle, vocation, relationships, status, possessions, etc.)
- Can I love myself just as I am, regardless of my personal image, relationships, achievements, possessions or the opinions of others?
- Can I feel compassion for myself and other human beings, without having a reason to do so?
- What does self-love look like to me? Does it sometimes take material form, like new clothing, a sweet treat or glass of wine? Or is it a deeper experience of kindness and care?

Having answered these questions as fully as you can, see if you can practise this first part of the loving-kindness meditation for more than ten minutes:

- Find a comfortable sitting position and allow your mind to settle by beginning to focus on your breathing.

- Take a moment to reflect on yourself.
- Spend some time generating compassion for yourself in all your human-ness.
- After five or ten minutes, you may want to include your baby in this and cultivate love for both of you.

Great Expectations

Expectations and desired outcomes for birth can become a focal point towards the end of pregnancy, and on one hand it is really helpful to believe in our abilities, and to have a positive image of how we want to be in labour and birth, or of how we want our labour and birth to be. However, our wishes can also create pressure, influencing our desire to control what happens. The human will for security struggles when it is in the 'unknown zone', and we strive to manifest the future we want by becoming attached to the 'right' outcome.

But the more we become attached to possible future outcomes, the less present we are to what *is*. And actually being in this moment at every opportunity during the lead-up to the birth may bring more calm into our lives than potentially planting a seed of anxiety around wanting a specific kind of birth, or disappointment in the possibility of this not happening. We need not dismiss our expectations, but rather hold them in our awareness by choosing to witness them with compassion instead of judgement. Expectations for the birth might derive from our ideas of what is best or safest or most comfortable, or from other people's suggestions about how birth should be, which may all be completely valid. And we can do our best as mothers to prepare for childbirth, both inwardly and outwardly. There will also be influences in labour that we can try to manage, to give ourselves the very best conditions for birth. But ultimately labour and birth will unfold in their own way, which could surpass, reach or fall short of our expectations.

Being Open to What Is
One of the greatest contributions to enabling a woman to have a natural birth is if she has a safe, loving space to labour without interference, at her own pace. And yet even this cannot ensure a given result – which is why being open to 'what is' can be so freeing, because the energy we would otherwise be putting into our expectations is released so we can become present to just 'being'.

My feeling is that we need to trust ourselves and to trust in our birth process. We can try to create optimum conditions for birth, by preparing ourselves (and our birth partners) in alignment with our best intentions, and this is great. Know what you want, find examples of methods and positions to help your body do what it can do (also see resources section), and hold it all lightly rather than tightly. Try using your mindfulness practice to support your ability to be open in all ways. Birth is all about opening up.

THINGS PEOPLE SAY

During the perinatal year, parents will almost certainly at some point encounter the judgements, beliefs or stories of others, whether solicited or not. And while many of these will celebrate and affirm birth, babies and our parental path, not all will be supportive.

It is a mother who is likely to receive more comments and offerings – from medical attendants, family, friends, acquaintances, even bystanders. Someone might share a difficult birth story without invitation; or a care provider might inadvertently make negative or unsubstantiated statements about mother or baby. Things can be said thoughtlessly that can then unnecessarily occupy us with thoughts of fear or failure. But what we choose to do with this information will either empower or disempower us.

If we move into a state of deeper self-awareness during meditation, and notice our own responses to such incidents, we can begin to recognize the thoughts and emotions evoked and find acceptance for them. Mindfully looking at the comments of others can help us to consider them not necessarily as statements of truth but as judgements or stories created from someone else's anxiety, will to control or expressions of their own unresolved experience.

Unless we are being offered sound medical advice based on unequivocal diagnosis (and even then we can seek a second opinion), it is generally good not to take on negative projections from others, but to find the inner strength to create compassionate boundaries around our own self-belief and be *open* to our own experience – which is all that matters.

GOING INTO YOUR PRE-BIRTH CAVE

◆

*The last month or so of pregnancy asks you to find calm and solitude.
External stimuli may feel less important, social gatherings may seem
irrelevant, and you might be wanting to cosy up at home a lot. Your
quiet cave is calling you.*

IT IS NATURAL FOR HEAVILY PREGNANT WOMEN to forget
things, to lack concentration and to decline party invita-
tions. This is because a pre-birth mother is physically getting
ready for her own event, the importance of which far out-
weighs anything else happening in her vicinity. Hormonally,
she is tuning in to parts of her brain that might not be so
matter-of-fact. She is nesting and she may need to zone out of
other people's energies and fall back into her own quietude.

I like to think of it as a 'closing in' time, when only the
simple bare necessities matter. A phase when you can justifi-
ably close your door to the world in the knowledge that it will
still be there when you re-emerge later on, as you attend to
the wonderful task of just *being* in readiness for birth. This is
also a perfect moment to meditate, and if your meditation
becomes sleep, welcome it! Especially if you are experiencing
phases of insomnia or other distractions from sleep at night,
such as frequent urination. Every opportunity to rest and
rejuvenate is good, so try to devise ways of having a regular
daily meditation or nap time.

Rest is Never Wasted

Rest, in the last days of pregnancy, is never wasted. Notice when you want to stop and meet your needs as best you can. You can bring mindfulness into these moments by watching your breath, noticing your thoughts and feelings and the sensations in your body, and just by bringing in acceptance for all you are experiencing.

The cumulative effect of unwinding pre-labour will benefit you greatly when labour actually begins, as you will be better resourced with fresh energy for what lies before you. Honour your body's gradually increasing secretion of oxytocin by doing things that support it, like cuddling, laughing and, closer to the time of birth, lovemaking (the high levels of oxytocin secreted in us as we make love can initiate labour, so it is best not to shake the tree too much before the apples are ripe, so to speak). But just be kind to this extraordinary woman that you are, about to bring a new life into this world. You deserve for your needs to be met.

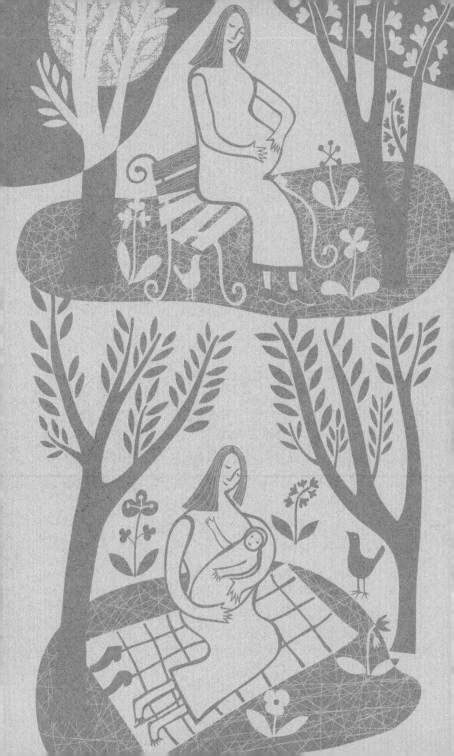

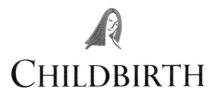

CHAPTER THREE

CHILDBIRTH

*Both mystery and miracle meet with physiology
and science in the epic journey of childbirth. A mother
facilitates this life-giving event with her powerful and
sophisticated body. It is truly an act of faith, courage
and love, both sacred and unpredictable. It is our
mothers' greatest gift to us, and in turn, their mothers'
greatest gift to them, all the way back through our
female lines. And as we venture into birth, we touch
the spiritual substance of welcoming a new
life to Earth.*

BIRTH IS A PROCESS

◆

The experience of labour and birth will vary widely from woman to woman. It is a process that requires our dedicated focus and self-belief and our body's deep permission and surrender. But, ultimately, birth will find its own rhythm in us.

I SOMETIMES THINK THAT IF THE BUDDHA had been a mother, or if there had been a substantial number of Buddhist teachers who were mothers since his time, there would be plenty of ancient teachings on the practice of meditation during labour. In fact, it would probably have been seen as the perfect opportunity for attaining insight, wisdom and even enlightenment – because, in many ways, it is.

All the ingredients for *being with what is* – at its most intense – can be found in birth. It is a physical experience that asks us to feel all of its sensations, while hormonally, emotionally and spiritually we are primed for entering into a heightened state of consciousness, which can somehow help us to go beyond everything we feel. During labour, our body's natural feel-good endorphins, alongside oxytocin and prolactin – which create blissful feelings – are all at their zenith.

Our body's generous production of melatonin also invites us to relax, further enabling the secretion of oxytocin. This is *the* most hormonally powered moment in our entire lives, with the potential to take us to a place of profound love and awakening. Perhaps it is this aspect of childbirth that calls women to do it again, or perhaps it is just because babies are so beautiful, or because pregnancies happen. But in all cases the pull of love can keep this experience alive in us forever.

Oxytocin's Leading Role

Oxytocin is quite simply the central hormone that progresses labour towards birth, and its presence is synchronous with feelings of love and care. We experience it throughout our lives, but it peaks in childbirth to a much, much higher degree than at any other time. We secrete this hormone when our hearts are open, when we are joyfully relaxed and laughing, and when we are sexually active. In women, oxytocin is also secreted in combination with prolactin (the 'mothering' hormone) towards the moment of birth, and through motherly, loving connections with babies and children, especially breastfeeding, skin-to-skin and physical closeness. Massage also prompts the release of oxytocin and even loving words, gazing into a lover's eyes or kissing can spark it into action.

A Sensual Experience

Seeing birth as an oxytocin-rich experience sets the scene for how we might want it to be for us. Feeling loved and supported by those around us is important, as are physical touch, compassion, encouragement and a relaxed environment. But it is also valuable to know that sensual and sexual contact with your partner positively affects your labour and birth by stimulating and maintaining your body's oxytocin levels.

Having private time with your lover can help to restart a stalled labour, and keep labour's momentum going. It is beautiful to think that the body chemistry surrounding a child's conception is the same as that which will facilitate their birth, and it is empowering for couples to embrace this approach if it feels right. You can include the option to have uninterrupted private time with your partner in your birth preferences, so that if you have been disturbed by anything in labour and need to calmly return to your birth focus, this is much easier to do.

SURRENDER TO THE BODY

The vast power of the female body becomes enshrined in the act of childbirth. In the 'ideal' design of things, the beautiful life created in the safe and perfect container of our womb passes through our pelvis, birth canal and vagina, miraculously defying the size of this orifice, to become another amazing, individual body.

OUR BODIES ARE AMAZING, and we can feel great awe for ourselves in gestating a baby, and birthing one (or more than one!), even if our birth route does not resemble the 'ideal' design. I feel I can put my hand on my heart and say it was my body that gave birth to my children. All I could do was to continue allowing it to do the work it was already doing, and I was humbled by its extraordinary abilities. Once I was in the saddle of labour, it took me with it and I surrendered to wherever it had to go.

It is so beneficial for us to learn to trust our bodies. To listen to them and respect what they tell us, because they are the ones who know how to grow and birth our babies; who will tell us if something isn't right and who will show us what they need. It might sound strange to speak of our bodies as separate to ourselves, but an involuntary physical process, such as vomiting, is not something we can consciously control or 'do' but rather we allow it to happen and support it. Things inside or outside of us might influence, stimulate or diminish the process, but it will occur of its own accord.

So exploring being in your body in pregnancy is very good preparation for birth – feeling into where you may need extra support, or what is comfortable for you and what is not. Trying positions you feel might work for you in labour is also really helpful. I have only given birth on all fours with my upper body slightly raised, which meant that I couldn't actually see either of my babies being born, but I certainly felt them, like a force of nature moving through my entire being.

This position enables the pelvis to open up more than in any other birth posture, and having the chest tilted upwards onto a birth ball also engages the pull of gravity to bring the baby downwards. Women who use this posture are statistically more likely to give birth with their perineum intact.

MINDFUL EXERCISE

BIRTH MEDITATION PRACTICE

This exercise is intended to support you in mindfully and joyfully exploring physical movement. It is excellent preparation for birth and also wonderful for use in labour itself. Try it when you can be alone, and give yourself complete permission to let go and move as you want, just enjoying being in your body. Remember to stay within your physical limits and not to push or overstretch yourself.

- Dim the lights or close the curtains and put on some music that inspires and relaxes you. The dimming of light supports our body's production of melatonin, while the music plays a fundamental role by stimulating the hypothalamus, which aids the secretion of essential birth hormones, thus deepening our connection with our own inner birth 'state' and helping our body to function at an optimum.

- Now explore how your body feels being on all fours or in a lateral position. You can also experiment with a birth ball, chair or bed to lean on, which can be especially good if you have swollen or painful wrists. You may want to see how it feels to have cushions under your belly to relieve the weight, and under your knees too.

- Once you have found a good position, start to become aware of the flow of your breathing, in and out.

- Notice the sensations in your body and what stands out to you most — perhaps areas of weight pulling down, or the pressure of contact with what is beneath you, or any tightness in your muscles.

- As you become more present to the feelings in your body, try to let go and relax a little more in any areas of tension, and continue to follow your breath in and out.

- Then gradually start exploring small movements such as rocking, swaying or very gently arching, flexing and rolling your spine. Notice if your breath changes as you move.

- Give yourself complete permission to listen and follow your body's urges to move, without self-judgement. Fully engaging with the music can help you to do this.

- Keep returning to the flow of your breathing.

- If you are holding any tension in your mouth, jaw or throat, try to stretch out and release it. Softening your jaw muscles also helps to relax the muscles in your pelvic area, cervix and birth canal, so practising this is very helpful for labour. Sense what you find in your body as you do this.

- Keep moving and allow yourself to be really present in your body by noticing your breath and physical sensations.

- Perhaps try to forget about time if you can and keep going for as long as you wish to.

- When you are ready to complete this exercise, just sit in relaxation for a little while and journal about how it felt.

- Try to practise this exercise regularly before the birth to develop your joyful connection with movement and become more familiar with physically letting go.

The only way to make sense

out of change,

Is to plunge into it,

Move with it,

And join the dance.

FROM 'THE WISDOM OF INSECURITY'
ALAN WATTS (1915–1973)

Joyful Movement in Birth

As a way of shifting from the neocortex, thinking-focused part of our brain and into deeper states of a more body-connected consciousness before labour, I encourage pregnant women to spend time listening to music that inspires them, to feel into it and to move however they want to, embodying their dance instinctively. Since my first child was born I have seen labour and birth as a dance. I danced through both my pregnancies and labours and for many years have held dance spaces for pregnant women.

I believe it can benefit us so much to be physically 'fluid' in labour and to be completely authentic in our self-expression and self-permission in movement. By dance, I do not mean a performance, but quite the opposite. You could say that it is more like authentic movement that originates from deeply listening to your body and is also inspired by music. Your labour-dance can be approached with eyes closed in dim light with no one watching, and it might not look like anything you have done before, especially not like dancing. But it is a practice that encourages us to find the joy in moving, in rhythm and in being a physical body.

Self-Consciousness

It can take courage to be physically 'free' in labour, especially if you feel self-conscious of others watching you. If you are not worried by what others think, so much the better, but if you are, then it may be possible for your birth partner to arrange for you to be alone together, or for you to be on your own if you prefer that. If you are at home, your midwife can sit in the next room, or if you are in hospital your birth partner can usually arrange this, unless you are undergoing medical intervention that requires staff to be present.

Self-consciousness triggers the neocortex part of our brain, which can then slow labour down because it interferes with the process of hormonal secretion governed by the hypothalamus at the base of our skull. Privacy also plays a central role during the initial dilation stage of labour because the cervix is the largest sphincter in the body and it behaves very much like those of the anus and the urethra, whereby it will not open easily in the presence of strangers.

Find the joy in moving, in rhythm and in being a physical body

◆

Excretory, cervical and vaginal sphincters
function best in an atmosphere of intimacy and
privacy ... where interruption is unlikely or impossible.
These sphincters cannot be opened at will. When a
person's sphincter is in the process of opening, it may
suddenly close down if that person becomes upset,
frightened, humiliated or self-conscious.

FROM 'INA MAY'S GUIDE TO CHILDBIRTH'
INA MAY GASKIN

◆

Becoming aware of our self-consciousness is also useful; noticing when you feel it and what it brings up for you. It can be an experience of shyness, embarrassment or even fear. If it is a significant feeling for you, it may relate to past events having left traces of trauma and emotion. Sexual abuse can also impact on how safe we feel in pregnancy, as our whole reproductive system is being activated by growing a baby in our womb. In truth, pregnancy and birth hold the potential to become an amazing process of emotional and physical healing for us all, even for the most difficult feminine wounding such as this. However, we may need the support of deep-reaching therapeutic work to help this happen. Focusing on the breath to release stress at difficult moments also helps, and again, cultivating self-compassion is so important in creating an inner sense of love and safety.

Feeling Safe in Birth

All human beings have a need for privacy at times, some of us more so than others. But there could not be a more crucial time for a woman to have privacy than during the birth of her children, and sometimes disrupting this quiet space can interfere with the flow of labour. An uninterrupted labour is more likely to create the best conditions for a woman's body to do all it can for her to birth her child. But there may be times during labour when our private space *is* interrupted, and this can have an effect both physically and psychologically. So how can we meet challenges like this in the intense space of birth?

This is a wide area because there are so many possibilities surrounding each woman's desires for birth, including place of birth and who will be attending it. For some women, being in a hospital will feel safer, while for others it may be that having a doula present, or being in a pool at home, is more reassuring. Touch back to the section about your expectations for birth and reflect on what these are, then ask yourself if it would be possible for you to feel safe with whatever unfolds for you in birth. This is powerful preparation for childbirth because it prompts us to consider how we could meet *what is* in a situation that we cannot know in advance.

Cultivating self-compassion is so important in creating an inner sense of love and safety

Exploring our Inner Territory

If we have done as much as we can prior to birth to ensure we are surrounded by good birthing conditions, then perhaps the last remaining territory to survey is the inner one. Ask yourself, 'Can I be clear about my needs and wants in labour? Yet can I simultaneously be open to other possibilities that could happen or be necessary, and still feel safe in myself?' We can spend time beforehand exploring our feelings about potential variables in labour, naming and making space for these, and we can consider the kinds of responses we might have to them if they happened.

STRESS-SENSITIVE SYSTEMS

Jane Hardwicke Collings, Australian midwife, author and facilitator of women's workshops, speaks of our hormonally steered female rhythms, those guiding menstruation and childbirth especially, as being 'stress-sensitive' systems. She states that women will notice anxiety, irritation and inner challenges at these power points in our cycles so much more when we are living with stress. Conversely, love, relaxation and calm are the most positive influences on childbirth, and to be able to bring these qualities into our birth experience we need to have a relationship with them first. Having a birth partner who is committed to protecting and supporting a loving and gentle environment around us is also an invaluable asset.

Yet the most profound impact could come through using a mindfulness approach to just be in this moment, becoming aware of any anxiety or hopes around feeling safe that arise in us during these explorations. Continuing to be present right now, accepting how we feel and tuning in to a quality of safety inside ourselves is one positive way to approach whatever lies ahead. And in cultivating compassion for ourselves as women about to experience one of the biggest events of our lives, we can imbue this sense of safety with self-love and acceptance.

Out of our personal practice we can then bring self-care, curiosity and presence into birth and use them to ride the waves of labour, as it happens, so that if fear arises it can be embraced in the holding space of our awareness rather than magnified in our minds by panic. This is also relevant to our experience physiologically, because fear causes muscles to tense up and contract, making it more likely that labour will be painful. And by instigating the production of stress hormones as well, every physical effect of fear is at odds with the body's needs for labour.

The Witness in Labour

◆

Meditation practice does not have to involve sitting or lying. It can be used in any situation, and can be approached just as a way of experiencing things. We can apply this to being in labour and use our awareness as a compassionate container for our whole experience.

As a doula, I support women and couples through pregnancy and birth in a non-medical capacity. In this role, I would never ask a labouring woman to become more mindful of her experience. The willingness to practise mindfulness in childbirth has to come from her, otherwise it could feel patronizing or take her out of her own process. If she is already engaged with all of her focus in her own experience, then she is fully present to it. And mindfulness can happen spontaneously in labour, especially if we have a relationship with this practice already.

The gift of bringing a mindful approach into labour, however, lies in the ability to defuse negative reactions to what we may be feeling physically. If we become aware of any inner stories that could be escalating the belief that we 'can't do it' or that 'it is too much', and just watch these reactions rather than run with them, it is possible for us to create an anchor of calm for ourselves. Beyond this, we can guide our conscious awareness back to our body without letting our mind's judgements rule the way we perceive the sensations present in us.

My Memory of Childbirth

To explore this, I would like to share a simple observation that comes from my experience of giving birth for the first time, which I hope may be helpful in bringing more relaxation into your own birth process. Let's begin with some important terminology: in labour, our bodies are steeped in sensations – let's call this physical, sensing aspect the 'Feeler'. Then we also have the inner-thinker, who might judge and react to these sensations, whom we will call the 'Thinker',

A mindful approach to labour can defuse negative reactions

and lastly we have the 'Witness', who watches all of this internally. In order to describe how these factors can interrelate in labour, I will recount to you what I remember.

I was really keen to give birth for the first time and was excited when labour finally started, in the comfort of my own home. Even though my early labour was quite intense, I enjoyed the contractions and, as I mentioned earlier, I danced my way through the first few hours, really welcoming every wave of energy as it rushed through my body. As time wore on, though, I started to feel tired and the surges became very powerful, accompanied by equally strong sensations. This phase seemed to go on forever and, as we neared midnight, I began to question my capacity to keep going. It was so much more full-on than I had anticipated, but neither could I give up.

How Much Longer?

Although our affirmation for this birth was the word 'YES!', which my husband uttered during each contraction, the Thinker aspect of me became activated and I began having fearful thoughts and wondering how much longer I would be in labour. My Thinker wanted to know how dilated I was in an attempt to work this out, yet my internal experience moved between exploring the sensations of each surge with the curiosity of the Witness, and judging them.

At some point in the early hours of the morning, it was as though the waves that had been crashing through my body finally took me with them and I no longer felt the same kind of fear about them, even though they became more intense than before. This was during the transition stage, as I began to push my baby out. I felt ferocious, purposeful and more awake during each surge. I sensed every exquisite sensation of these powerful contractions and again, there I was: in the feelings, judging the feelings and simultaneously witnessing them.

I remember becoming aware that there was no turning back as my daughter's body moved down and through my birth canal... the only way was out! In the deep birth trance I was now in, nearly drifting off to sleep between the last few contractions, this almost came as a surprise to me. There is no other experience like a baby's head crowning at your vagina. Some women call it the ring of fire and often this moment does bring fear with it and it did for me too briefly, but I was able to let it go. The following contraction was a massive involuntary push in which my little baby girl flew out in one go and I was barely grazed by her body passing through me and into the world.

Sensation, Sensation, Sensation

Let's look at the relationship between the Feeler, the Thinker and the Witness in this process. My Feeler was experiencing sensations that I had never before encountered. All new and extremely strong, overwhelmingly so at times. My Thinker was gradually creeping into a place of fear and doubt, concerned about my well-being and trying to alert me to and protect me from pain, which is natural. My Witness, on the other hand, was completely present to my Feeler, fascinated by everything I was feeling because it was so huge and intense. And often they all blurred into one.

As I look back at this unique event in my life, I can see how much the awareness raised by my inner witness enabled me to accept my physical experience of childbirth without giving myself over to fear. All my previous yoga, dance and meditation practice had helped me to connect with my body as a feeler and listener, rather than by simply reacting to its sensations. And I know that when I was able to experience my Witness during the labour, I felt calmer and more *with* my body – so without 'doing' anything, I could be present to what was happening within me.

Everything in our body's chemistry allows us to go deeper into an extraordinary state of being during labour, with increasingly less emphasis on our critical thought processes. Knowing how many centimetres dilated we are does not help us to dilate more efficiently; nor will it necessarily give us an accurate description of our labour's duration, as the cervix can open quickly at times and less so at others. It only stops us from being present. And it stimulates the thinking mind, disrupting our connection with the hypothalamus part of our brain. So the more we can avoid this analytical, judgemental perception of our birth experience, the better for our body.

A FIRST TIME FOR EACH BIRTH

Four and a half years after the arrival of my first child, during the birth of my second, I discovered that each and every labour and birth is unique. I remember imagining that it would be the same kind of experience, but it couldn't have been more different.

My FIRST LABOUR WAS A POWERFUL and intense home birth that lasted about 14 hours. And while my second labour was also at home, it was gentle, with mostly 2 to 4 minutes between surges throughout, and entirely free of discomfort, except for the final few pushes. So even though I anticipated feeling the same as I had the first time around, I just didn't – not even marginally similar.

What this did was to wake me up. I kept expecting one thing and finding something else in its place, so again I became really present to everything I experienced in my body. I began listening with deep curiosity to each tightening, to the feeling in my abdominal muscles and to the spaces in between. My greatest surprise was when I suddenly felt the urge to poo and after a sequence of four massive contractions, my little boy was born, within about an hour and a half of established labour.

When a woman has given birth once, subsequent labours can be quicker and easier, but this is not always the case. In some ways, the body of a woman who has given birth before is a very different female body. Besides this, we will have a physiological and conscious memory of giving birth, which can really help to smooth the pathway unless there has been previous birth trauma or caesarean birth, in which case giving birth vaginally the next time may require specific preparation around healing past experience.

Natural Training

As first-time mothers, we can be awe-inspired by the experience of birth because our bodies have never done this amazing thing, or felt this intensity of sensation before. It might be reassuring for a first-time mother to have another supportive mother around her during labour who knows what it can feel like and who can reaffirm her experience as being something 'normal', that they too have felt.

Birth is a time of power and surrender,

of beginnings and endings, of primordial feelings

and absolute novelty. Your personal birth story echoes

the stories of women since the beginning of humankind,

yet it can be entirely unique.

FROM 'MAGICAL BEGINNINGS, ENCHANTED LIVES'
DEEPAK CHOPRA

In some ways, menstruation can be seen as a woman's natural bodily birth preparation. Most women have been fertile since they were girls and have spent a fair amount of their lives in the cycle of their menstrual flow before they become pregnant. As my fellow doula, Kate Woods, says, this is a good amount of time to get to know how you feel when you have your period, to sense what your needs are, and to get accustomed to the physical sensations in your womb. It's also true that the first actual experience of birth can still take us straight into the realms of beginner's mind if we're willing to go there.

Beginner's Mind, Every Time

When birth is absolutely new to our bodies, we can meet it through all of our senses with this quality of newness and openness. And as we do this, it becomes easier to see the mind's internal judgements in the same way, rather than using them to create a discouraging or fearful narrative about our experience. But as I described earlier in the story of my second birth, it is still possible to use this approach even if we have given birth several times before, because each birth experience will be new to us, just as each child we give birth to will be unique. Meeting childbirth with the curiosity and keen listening of a 'beginner' or learner can bring the spaciousness of non-judgement and embracing what is.

THE CHILDBIRTH ENVIRONMENT

There are many potential contributing factors in a woman's experience of birth. But if her environmental influences during labour are positive and supportive, she will have the best opportunity to follow her body's natural process.

WE, AS MOTHERS, CAN TRY TO GIVE OURSELVES the most expansive possibility of enabling our bodies to fulfil their potential. But the responsibility for a satisfying and healthy experience of birth also falls on the shoulders of our care providers. If the environmental conditions around us are not at an optimum to suit our deeper needs in labour, this can affect us. The course of childbirth can also be prescribed by our baby's well-being during labour and ultimately the outcome will focus on prioritizing their health. Building trust in yourself and your baby and belief in your body's abilities will help you to feel strong throughout.

Tightenings, Surges, Rushes and Waves

Labour's amazing rhythm works in a sequence of muscular contractions and expansions, making our uterus and the muscles around it tighten and relax over and over again, which can result in a very deep feeling of relaxation in between each tightening. You can try this for yourself now if you like. Just tense up the muscles in your whole body – face, feet, hands, everywhere. And hold it. Then let go, relax and breathe. Do you feel more relaxed than you did before you started? During labour, we also have our inner reservoir of hormones and endorphins, relaxing us even more.

Nonetheless, contractions can be powerful and can trigger pain receptors in the brain, which may provoke resistance, making us want to fight our body's natural rhythm. But if we struggle against labour it becomes far more difficult and in truth, the only way is to go with its flow. Finding ways to explore this attitude of surrender is very valuable in pregnancy.

Being With Discomfort

Nancy Bardacke, midwife and founder of the Mindfulness Based Childbirth and Parenting programme in the US, uses a simple exercise to help pregnant women to practise *being* with discomfort in preparation for the surges of labour. She begins by asking them to hold ice cubes in their hand for a whole minute and, initially, to concentrate on and verbally express all the discomfort they are feeling. Then they repeat this exercise, but this time she asks the participants to focus entirely on watching their breath. The difference in their perception of sensation from holding the ice is usually completely different between the first and second stages of this activity.

Try this for yourself and see the difference in your responses. Use one hand first and then the other, so they each go from warm to cold once. You can experiment with this, too, by exploring the sensations in your hand without any judgements about them, as you watch your breath. Developing this kind of mindful relationship with how we perceive sensation will serve us wonderfully well in childbirth.

Three Areas to Support You in Labour

1. The Breath

Breathing bonds us to life. It is also a huge part of labour and can support us through every stage of the journey. Bringing awareness to the cycle of our inhalation and exhalation can keep us focused during and between contractions, which is such a powerful anchor for our thoughts. Physically also, long out-breaths work to diminish the residual build-up of lactic acid created by so much exercise in the muscles around our wombs. We can actually 'breathe it out' and, in so doing, reduce the potentially uncomfortable cramping or feeling of 'runner's stitch' in areas of the lower body. It is really helpful to explore your breathing in using mindful awareness and counting is also a great focus for the mind.

COUNTING THE LENGTH OF A BREATH

Practise breathing in for four counts and out for eight to explore a cycle of breathing with longer exhalations. You can also ask your birth partner to count out loud for you if you want their support to help you keep focused on your breath. Remain aware of how you are breathing in labour. Ask yourself if your breath is supporting your birth process. If it is not, find a way of breathing that calms and centres you.

SOUNDING

Making steady, deep sounds in labour is a wonderful way of using your breath. From my personal experience, and from that of many women I have worked with, making effortless groaning sounds with the out-breath can also help to channel the intensity of each surge 'out' of the body. Rest into the power of your breath and sounds, and let them carry you.

2. The Body

POSITIONS

Your body is your vehicle in labour. Being comfortable in your body is really important and can ease physical strain and potential discomfort. Take the initiative to move and find positions that work for you. Certain postures can be used to gain the full effect of gravity, increasing the pressure of your baby against your cervix to assist dilation and helping the baby descend through the birth canal.

In labour, prepare your birth partner to ask you every now and then if you are in a good position and keep experimenting until you find an effective posture, changing it as you need to.

TOUCH

Other postures can provide access for your birth partner to massage your back or legs. The right kind of physical touch, massage, and pressing certain acupressure points are excellent natural analgesics and can be very reassuring to your body and mind, as well as encouraging the flow of oxytocin.

WATER

Being in warm water will lessen the effectiveness of gravity, but will soothe tired muscles, physical discomfort and emotional stress. Many women receive great support from immersion in water during labour and birth because it is naturally analgesic and physically nurturing and allows freedom of movement.

MOVEMENT

Movement can be very helpful. Circling the hips, rocking, swaying, pulling down on something above you, squatting, and other kinds of movement can all be used to reduce discomfort. By exploring movement in labour, we can listen and actively respond with our bodies to our own physical process, which is so empowering.

3. Relaxation

Being able to relax in childbirth is fundamental to the whole journey. Being aware of this during labour will guide you to discover ways of relaxing more. Asking yourself 'Where can I let go of tension in my body?' and 'How can I relax deeper into my birth state?' can prompt you to unravel any stress and find more ease in your experience. If you feel something is holding you back, or that you are resisting your labour, see if you can use your breathing to move through that barrier, to let go and surrender.

AFFIRMATIONS

Using birthing affirmations about your wonderful progress and your amazing capability can work to focus the mind positively. The 'YES!!!' mantra is great for welcoming everything in your experience and all that you are. It functions to both empower us and help us surrender in birth. Create at least one simple affirmation that you and your birth partner can use to bring calm and positivity to your labour.

MUSIC

Music really can relax us and help us to connect with our bodies, so it is a wonderful tool for unwinding more into labour. Create a playlist for birth. Make sure this is portable so that if you go into hospital, it can still help to maintain your relaxation levels in transit and throughout labour.

INTIMACY

If need be, ask everyone to leave the room so you can be alone to be intimate with your partner, if this is right for you.

ENVIRONMENT

Dim lighting and darkness help labour to progress as they support our production of melatonin, which both relaxes us and causes the womb to contract efficiently. Warmth is also important as it enables our muscles to soften and relax, and mother and baby must especially be kept warm after the birth.

Ask your birth partner to try to establish a sense of relaxation in your environment. Feeling uneasy or unsafe can lead to physical tension, which can result in pain. If something or someone in your environment is causing you to feel tense, ask your birth partner or doula to try to remedy this situation if possible. Prioritize your own relaxation and peace of mind because this will be continually informing your body that you are safe and supporting your progress throughout labour.

BIRTH PREFERENCES

You can put into writing any ideas you have around safeguarding your experience of labour in the areas outlined here, and add them to your birth preferences. This tells your care-provider about who you are and what you want and if your wishes are transgressed at any time, you can redirect your birth attendants to these written guidelines.

WELCOMING YOUR BABY

The moment your baby is born is truly special. This first meeting with your child after so many months of anticipation can bring joy, relief, surprise – and the indelible clarity of big new beginnings.

F OR SOME MOTHERS, the love affair with their baby really starts in this instant, while for others, there may be so much going on within and around them that the relationship can take a little more time to develop. Nevertheless, many, many women experience a feeling of falling in love as they gaze upon the face or into the eyes of their beloved new baby and it is a mysterious, suspended time of discovery and heart-opening that words cannot capture.

It is also an important bonding stage in the whole mother-baby journey, when breastfeeding can be initiated. Depending on the place of birth, there may be many ongoing distractions from this; however, the nuzzling of a newly born baby's face against your skin as they root for a nipple to begin suckling is a vital part of establishing their immune system. Receiving skin-to-skin contact directly after birth with you, or your partner, enables your baby to 'breathe' you in.

As they are inhaled, the microbes from your skin begin to colonize your baby's gut and create a healthy microbiome that will protect them for a lifetime. Vaginal birth also hugely increases the richness and diversity of microbes they absorb,

```
SLOWING DOWN
```

The post-birth bonding phase is key to creating a reassuring, safe welcome for your child, both emotionally and biologically, and it is worth protecting. Wherever you give birth, you can specify in your birth preferences that you would like things to slow down after your baby is born. This is usually possible, unless there are any complications. You may want to request an unhurried atmosphere in the room so you can fully focus on your baby. Depending on the country you give birth in, and the policies held by the hospital or birth centre you use, you can arrange for everything to be kept calm and quiet after the birth.

but even with a caesarean birth, your baby can be 'seeded' with your microbes to help boost their emerging immunity (see reference section for details). Breastfeeding also provides your baby with the enrichment of colostrum, a health-giving first milk-like substance that combines immune-assisting properties with more mother-borne microbes to generate the healthiest internal environment possible for your baby's body.

Labour's Third Stage

Post-birth, your care providers will have several require-ments to fulfil. One is to clamp your baby's umbilical cord. In general medical practice, this is usually done just after birth and before the cord has finished pulsating and carrying the remainder of nourishing blood from the placenta to the baby. However, there is much recent evidence showing far better outcomes for babies if clamping is postponed for a minimum of 3–5 minutes after birth so that they can receive the final third of their body's full quota of blood from the placenta. Some parents choose to leave the cord for up to 30 minutes before cutting it and some request a 'lotus birth', where the cord is left intact and later the placenta is preserved with salt, placed in fabric and kept with their baby until the cord naturally dries and detaches itself from baby's belly.

After birth, a mother will be tuning in to the needs of her baby

Another practical task is to check the baby's well-being and to administer vitamin K, either by injection or eye drops. This prophylactic is routinely carried out after birth to help prevent the extremely rare appearance of vitamin K deficiency bleeding. This intervention is optional and parents can choose whether they want it for their child or not. Your medical support team will also want to weigh your baby.

And finally, delivery of the placenta. This can take a little time and although some care providers want the placenta delivered as quickly as possible after the baby, often using a Syntocinon injection to instigate a medically managed third stage, it is again something you can negotiate. If you want to deliver the placenta naturally, at your own pace, you should be able to ask for that.

The Golden Hour

The 'golden hour' is a term given to creating the gentlest possible first hour of your child's life, which, if everything is normal, can be kept free from distractions and interruptions so you and your baby can fall in love. For parents who would rather keep all activity to a minimum after the birth, just to be really present with their little one, it can be possible to arrange for immediate skin-to-skin, to postpone weighing, washing and vitamin K, to delay the clamping of the cord or to have a lotus birth, and to take time, even up to an hour, to deliver the placenta naturally. If your midwife or obstetrician wants to check your baby, but you would like your baby to be skin-to-skin with you, they may be able to check him while he lies on you rather than on a table. Again, if this is discussed in advance with your care provider's agreement and written into your birth intentions, it can happen.

Presence

A mother may be very tired after childbirth. She may feel ecstatic, disorientated, sore, shaky, emotional, deeply relieved, or something else entirely. She will probably be hungry and thirsty. If she has had a caesarean birth without experiencing labour, she may feel more detached from the birth and be trying to adjust to it all, which can take time. But however she births, even as a mother is returning to herself after her own experience, which may have been huge, she will be tuning in to the needs of her babe. Pregnancy primes us hormonally and instinctually with this single-minded focus and labour can take these maternal features to their extreme.

Some medication used for pain relief in labour, such as Pethidine, or general anaesthetic for an emergency caesarean birth, dulls the senses and makes this post-birth time very sleepy for both mother and baby. General anaesthetic is only used in occasional instances and may at those times be unavoidable, but Pethidine is not a great option for pain relief because it affects your baby and slows down the whole bonding and feeding stage between you.

When you are alert, however, there is no other time like that of meeting one's child and the magical moments following this, when your baby is experiencing their first sensory feelings outside of the womb. If you can keep coming back to this embodied experience of being with your baby, regardless of what is going on around you, becoming present to each and every beautiful, felt subtlety of your first encounter with them, this will be likely to stay with you forever.

On Being a Mother

You are a mother. I honour you. It is a profoundly beautiful and also demanding path of service that you tread, so keep learning to honour yourself with each step of the way and let every part of this journey enable your heart to grow even bigger, to both give and receive.

If we lived now in the kind of cultures that many of our ancestors formed, thousands of years ago, mothers would no doubt feel the kind of pride that is derived from being revered as a goddess of fertility. I think I could get used to that, personally. But at this point in our evolution as a species, we have not yet remembered that gestation and birth are miraculous events in the abundant tides of creation on this planet. It is up to us to remember this for ourselves and to share it with those around us by embodying it.

If this sounds exaggerated, that is because we have become habituated to not seeing the sacredness of human life.

Motherhood is a physical, emotional, mental and spiritual process of transformation and to benefit fully from the personal revolution we undergo, we need to remain as open-hearted as we can to all of it, and to ourselves. Know that in being a mother you are doing something very special, even if this is not fully seen or acknowledged by others or by society. Let your personal understanding empower you and enable you to tread your path with self-respect, kindness and awareness. And if you don't already love yourself, let this journey take you there. Your children will show you the way.

◆

Oh what a power is motherhood.

EURIPIDES 480–406 BCE
ANCIENT GREEK DRAMATIST

◆

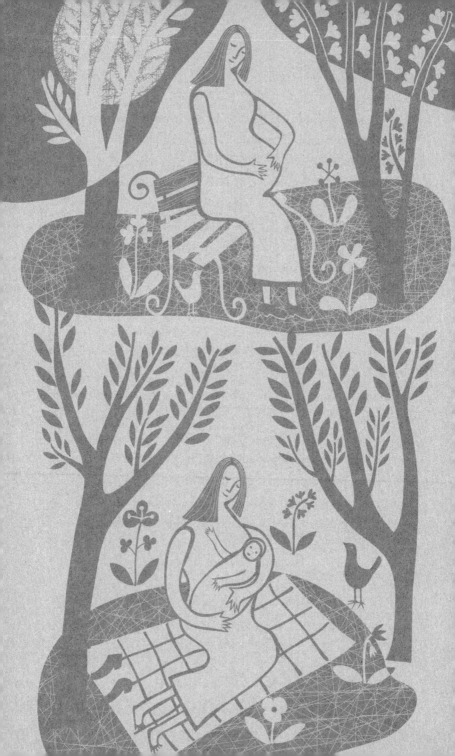

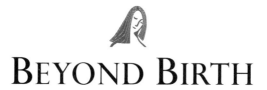

CHAPTER FOUR

BEYOND BIRTH

*We pass through birth's threshold, claiming
our child as the ultimate reward for our efforts, yet
the journey has just begun and we are travelling day
by day into the unknown with a newly born soul we
have still to discover. This is a multi-faceted phase,
filled with joy, intensity, exhaustion, beauty and many
varied experiences, feelings and sensations. Living in
the now, with acceptance and awareness of it all,
enables us to flow more with the ups and downs
of parenting in these early days.*

LIVING GENTLY WITH A NEWBORN

◆

Being gentle with ourselves after childbirth is very valuable, for both parents. We will be focused on meeting the needs of our little one as best as we can, but in order to give from a resourced place we also need to find nourishment, rest, patience and kindness for ourselves.

THE FIRST FEW WEEKS AFTER BIRTH can feel like a baby-moon, immersed in love, especially for a mother. For some, there will be interludes like this, but there may be challenges too. And many of us will face hurdles such as baby blues (discussed later), physical recovery from birth and taking on the huge responsibility of looking after a tiny baby. But it is such a profoundly love-filled time and it is vital to remember that the simpler we keep our lives during this stage, the easier and more enriched they will be.

This means keeping stress to a minimum because oxytocin is still playing a major role, facilitating the mother's process of bonding with her child, and a big part of this bond is developed through breastfeeding. The production of breast milk and breastfeeding itself, like a full circle of love, is also orchestrated by oxytocin, and prolactin. New mothers and babies who share these hormones through breastfeeding are literally LOVE-fuelled. But oxytocin is incompatible with stress hormones, so adding stress to this picture can affect a mother's milk supply and the ease with which she establishes feeding.

Why Breastfeed?

The benefits of breastfeeding are worthy of books dedicated entirely to them and if there was more public advertising about these, we would now be seeing a steeper rise in breast-feeding rates globally. But in brief, breastfed babies statistically cry less, have higher intelligence and significantly better immunity and are at less risk of infantile illnesses. They are also less likely to become obese or diabetic in the future.

A mother benefits from breastfeeding, too, as it reduces the chances of her developing post-natal depression or, later in life, going on to develop breast or ovarian cancer, diabetes or osteoporosis. Human breast milk is designed for a human baby and is far more digestible than other milks and better equipped to help them grow and develop. It is a much easier option than sterilizing bottles, teats and preparing formula milk. Feeding a baby by breast is also an ecologically ethical choice as it cuts out the environmental impact and waste of generating, packaging and distributing formula products.

Overcoming Difficulties

For some women, breastfeeding happens effortlessly and without discomfort. Yet many women who would like to breastfeed don't receive the best support or coaching that could help them to do so successfully and they assume or are told that they can't do it and should give up. If a mother becomes distressed by her difficulties with breastfeeding, obviously her well-being comes first and she has the option of feeding her baby with a bottle. However, she should be receiving the right kind of care and assistance from the beginning so that this kind of problem can be avoided.

Sadly, though, there are cultural or social reasons why a mother might not choose to breastfeed. In certain cases, it might not be physically possible; but, for example, having flat or inverted nipples will not stop you feeding and even a baby with an infantile condition such as tongue tie or cleft palate will still be able to feed from the breast with some professional measures in place to help. So if you have the support to hand, you can overcome most complications.

FREEDOM FROM GUILT

If a mother had intended to feed but decided for some reason to stop, this can bring up feelings of guilt and self-judgement, which are very heavy emotions to carry alongside the potential sleep deprivation and everything else she is managing. Becoming aware of any stories we create around feeding our babies may help us to make more space for cultivating self-kindness in our thoughts and feelings. It is so helpful to remember that we are human, we are fully supporting another dependent human life and we are doing the very best we can. We can only do our best and if the challenges that we face are too steep then we need to choose an easier way, preferably without strings of guilt attached.

Learning to Latch

If you are pregnant for the first time and want to breastfeed your baby, or are considering it, connect with other breastfeeding mums and find a breastfeeding group before you give birth, to observe and talk about how it is done. Find a good book to read about it, too (see reference section). Although it is a fairly straightforward task, there are some intricacies you need to grasp early on to ease the process. The longer you feed your baby as they grow, the easier it can become. But in the early stages an inexperienced mother will need guidance, and the first step to learn is the right positioning for the 'latch' – the secure suction of the baby's mouth onto your nipple and breast.

Relaxed breathing and self-kindness are the best guards against stress

I have known mothers who have tried to latch their babies onto the breast time after time without success, and have felt hopeless because of this. But unless we have grown up in a pro-breastfeeding culture, where mothers are doing it in private *and* in public, how do we learn about it? A breastfeeding expert once told me that more than a hundred latches in one sitting is fine when you are starting out, that both mother and baby are learning and this takes time. Stress is the most important element to avoid while acquiring the skill of breastfeeding as it impedes the milk flow, and relaxed breathing and self-kindness are the best possible guards against this.

Encourage yourself with every try and seek professional support if you want or need to. Breastfeeding a newborn can be uncomfortable to begin with. Even when you have a great position and your baby is latched on securely, it can feel sore for a week or two while your nipples are adjusting to their new job. But if you can master a good latch technique it does get much easier, and soon the oxytocin released during each feed brings such overwhelmingly loving feelings with it that it can become the highlight of both a mother and baby's day! I breastfed over the course of two years and every moment I spent feeding were the most rewarding and uplifting of all that I can recall during that precious time with my babies.

Support for Discomfort and Stress

If feeding is painful for you in these early days, this can generate anxiety and even distress. Feelings like this can be intensified if your baby cries a lot, as our maternal instinct is to feed and comfort, yet doing so might bring discomfort. If this is your second or third baby or more, you may also have the intense experience of your womb contracting back to size with every feed you give. The discomfort of this can be counteracted by using a tens machine for the few days that it lasts. But if you are experiencing any kind of stress or physical problems around breastfeeding your baby, connect with someone who has professional experience in helping mothers and babies to feed, and try to find several sources of support.

MINDFUL EXERCISE

TREAT YOURSELF WITH KINDNESS

Besides seeking assistance from others when we are having difficulties with breastfeeding, we can work inwardly and mindfully by tuning in to our experience and exploring.

- **The breath** How is my breathing right now? Can I relax it more?
- **The sensations** What am I feeling in my body? Can I relax into these sensations a little more? (Notice if you have aversion to meeting any discomfort and just breathe into this feeling.)
- **The thoughts** What thoughts or beliefs arise for me as I am feeding or am about to feed my baby?
- **The feelings** What feelings are behind these thoughts or beliefs? Can I welcome these feelings with compassion, so that I can befriend myself and all my vulnerabilities even more?

When we bring compassion and relaxation to a place of suffering, we invite it to transform. In this space, our breath and physical tension can soften and the emotional intensity we feel can begin to ease. This is a very valuable remedy for the sometimes extreme landscape of a new parent's world.

Every attempt you make to breastfeed is a step along the loving path of nurturing your baby. Be as kind to yourself as you can possibly be. It may take time and there may be physical obstacles to overcome, but it is very likely that you will succeed. And if ultimately it is not possible, for whatever reason, keep being kind to yourself and know that you are still an amazing mother doing your very best you can for your child. Try to connect with these compassionate feelings for yourself, even in the midst of any self-judgements or feelings of disappointment that might arise.

From Colostrum to Breastmilk

The term 'baby blues' doesn't refer to post-natal depression, but to a short phase lasting for several days when a mother's milk comes in. After having produced colostrum for two or three days since the birth, the hormonal surge that causes us to suddenly start making milk almost universally brings tears with it. The majority of women have this experience and it makes us emotional, and is absolutely normal. It is good to be aware that this will happen and that you can use mindfulness tools to guide you through this stage without falling into any judgements or assumptions about the emotions themselves.

One easy and helpful technique is to use the phrase 'I am experiencing ...' and just list all the sensations, feelings and thoughts about your experience that stand out to you. It can also help to say these things out loud so you can hear yourself speaking them, as this can bring another perspective to each

FEELING LOW LONGER TERM

If the blues persist for weeks, or you have a sense of emotional numbness around your baby, please look into the possibility of receiving extra support. There are organizations, listed in the reference section at the back of this book, who specialize in helping women post-birth with symptoms of depression. It takes courage to reach out, but you and your baby will benefit so much in the long run from making this choice.

of your experiences. If you do this, try not to judge yourself or your words as you speak, but wholeheartedly welcome them, honouring your courage to work with yourself in this way.

You may want to return to the phrase 'I am experiencing' whenever you are in the midst of an internal struggle or are feeling confused or are too tired to think straight. It has a way of engaging the mind with the simple, momentary phenomenon you may be facing, in a way that is calming and centring and cultivates self-acceptance.

HEALING BODY

Depending on her birth experience, a mother's body will be healing to different degrees after birth. But whatever our experience, when we consciously remind ourselves that we are a human mass of cellular regeneration in a constant process of healing, we confirm our body's progress.

AFTER MY FIRST CHILD, even though I had a natural vaginal birth and my perineum was intact, I felt as though my internal organs took their time to gradually settle back into place. My body felt askew and creaky and I couldn't stand fully upright for a few days. I also experienced discomfort as I breastfed my baby, which lasted a week or so. But the state of absolute baby-bliss I was in seemed to counteract any concern about my body, which I believe helped me to heal swiftly.

After my second birth, I felt physically more able but, because he was my second child, my womb vigorously contracted back to size as I breastfed (much more so than with a first child), making the experience more difficult. I also developed a cracked nipple early on because I assumed I could remember how to breastfeed without revision and didn't check our 'nose-to-nipple' positioning properly. This was sore, and meant I had to feed with one breast and express milk with the other for a day until, after applying lots of calamine ointment and keeping it open to the air, it had healed well enough to feed my baby again.

Hold That Thought

This being said, I know my own birth and post-birth experiences have been straightforward and easy in relation to some mothers', and that the whole journey can be a lot more physically challenging, especially if it involves recovery from exhaustion, surgery or infection. Holding the thought 'My body is healing' helps to frame this situation in a positive light, bringing hope even if we are feeling uncomfortable. It is also true that the cells in our bodies are renewing themselves incessantly from minute to minute and hour to hour.

However, it is also important to honour our bodies and our levels of discomfort and to reach out for support if we need it, rather than struggling through. It really is an act of self-compassion to prioritize our health, particularly as new mothers, when our body's natural healing time during sleep is disrupted by night waking. Being aware that our personal well-being will benefit the well-being of our baby, partner and family as a whole might help us to take it seriously.

Regular baths in warm water with an infusion or tincture of hypericum and calendula are great for healing the perineum after an episiotomy or tear, or for mothers recovering from a caesarean birth. Women normally bleed from the womb, as we would during our menses, for between one and six weeks after giving birth. But if the bleeding is heavy, again do seek medical advice as soon as you can.

Mindful Nutrition

It is also important for new mothers to be putting into their bodies more than they are putting out, so it is essential to eat a fresh, healthy and nourishing diet, rich in iron, protein and good unsaturated oils, with plenty of pure water. And teas taken daily, such as nettle, fennel, peppermint and fenugreek, are excellent in helping to boost or maintain a mother's milk supply if necessary.

Eating and drinking can also become opportunities for mindfulness meditation, as life will probably be very full with baby-caring. The act of chewing or sipping, swallowing and ingesting food and drink, with a focus on 'receiving' through the senses of smell, taste and touch, can create mindful spaces that might otherwise be lost in the tides of doing or sleeping.

And trying to do this with gratitude, and an intention to fully absorb and be nourished by what we take in, can enrich and deepen our relationship with the nutrition that sustains us.

Healing Heart and Mind

For some new mothers, it is more than the physical body that needs to heal after childbirth, especially if the experience has been traumatic or disappointing in some way. After giving birth, we may sometimes be left with the impression that our care provider did not offer what we needed in order for us to have a truly fulfilling birth experience. This can trigger feelings of regret, sadness, dissatisfaction and anger and lead us into a place of emotional 'stuckness' or resignation.

Some of us may feel that we, or our bodies, were 'unable' to give birth and there might be a sense of having let ourselves down, failing, inadequacy and shame; but I don't believe a mother fails when her birth doesn't go to plan. Experiencing childbirth, whatever the outcome, bears testimony to our courage and strength and we can claim self-love and respect from this same ground that might otherwise yield self-judgement and condemnation, if birth left us feeling inadequate, disempowered or numb.

But in all circumstances, the resulting emotions can be draining and difficult to bear when we have the demanding task of baby-rearing to handle, without being resourced with much sleep. It is important, for our own sakes, to find ways of integrating a challenging experience of birth. Being able to find peace in ourselves is not easy in a situation like this, but it will help us to thrive in every way if we do. It may be that time or therapeutic support is needed for the healing of our wounds. However, in the short term it may also be possible for us to connect with an inner place of peace in the moments when we are faced with thoughts that hook us into those depleting emotions and internal narratives.

Unpack Your Birth Story
Before attempting this, though, I would suggest taking a bit of uninterrupted time to unpack your birth story. You can do this by asking a trusted friend, relative or therapist to simply listen to you, without judgement, while you describe your experience of labour, part by part, expressing everything you felt and thought along the way. You can use a journal to download all of this if you prefer. When you have finished, try to make time to sit in meditation and cultivate some 'metta', or loving-kindness, for yourself and for your baby.

This exercise in itself will not necessarily help you to find more acceptance for what happened, and it is completely okay if it doesn't. But from this point onwards, try to notice when you are experiencing difficult thoughts, feelings or physical sensations related to your birth story. When you catch them rising up, just pause in the midst of them and return to your breath, become present to the sensations in your body, relax and release any tension. To deepen your relaxation, bring in a quality of compassion for yourself and all you have been through. The more you practise this regular, mindful engagement with peace and self-kindness, the more likely the negative emotional charge around your experience of birth will start to fade, allowing you to feel more spacious and available to the life you are leading here and now.

And practising self-care in this way doesn't stop you making a complaint or taking issue with your health-care provider if that is what is needed, but it means you can do so from a more centred and empowered place in your heart.

BABYMOON

As you turn down the volume of life so you can focus on this brief and beloved time with your baby as a newborn, you might like to think of it as a baby-holiday and take a rest from all your normal daily rituals and activities.

You are absolutely justified to forget about emails, telephones and television, to let weeds take over the garden and to stay in your pyjamas all day for weeks. You may also want to consider eliminating any tasks that might drain your energy. Even chores like going to the supermarket can be abandoned in favour of shopping online or asking a friend or relative to pick up groceries for you, or to bring a meal over. Frozen meals that you remembered to make before the birth also come in handy now (take note).

Putting off unwanted visits is also good – even if you feel under pressure to introduce your new baby to your inner circle, there is no need to do this if you are tired and don't feel like it. And if this brings up guilt, it represents another opportunity for self-enquiry and to affirm your compassionate boundaries around honouring your own needs above the expectations or projections of others. But if you do want to see people and invite them over, ask them to help by 'hosting' you, rather than you hosting them, and let them know when you need them to leave so you can rest.

Reducing stress is actually pivotal in creating a smoother passage throughout every aspect of family life, so now is the perfect stage just to bond with and delight in your baby above all else and to let go of anything that causes you stress or distracts you from this.

Rest
Living without the sustenance of a normal sleeping pattern is tricky, and this is usually how things are for parents, especially for breastfeeding mothers, in the first months of your baby's life. If sleep loss affects you very badly, you may want to try coordinating night shifts with your partner when you need a break, and expressing milk so that they can wake and feed the baby while you have a full night off. Even so, it is likely

that you will still have a sleep deficit and this can mount up incrementally, leading to low reserves later on.

I experienced a six-month burnout with both my children – while being deliriously infatuated with them, I couldn't cope with the intensive mothering and sleep deprivation combination, month after month. I went through a lull at about six or seven months when I felt as if I was actually delirious and I would have given anything for a good night's rest, or a week of them.

Having said that, I did breastfeed exclusively and they slept next to me every night without exception, until they were well over a year old. And they were not great sleepers, so nor was I. Being idealistic like me is fine but, in retrospect, if I had taken my own well-being into account, I could have enjoyed those first years more. I understand now how important this element of self-care is in the life of a mother, because if she over-extends herself, the whole family will feel it.

Ways to Prevent Burnout

To prevent this happening, try to rest whenever you can and even call in some help. Living in nuclear-style families is not really the natural way for child-rearing, as our community-dwelling ancestors understood so well, and it is such a help to have friends or family at hand if they are needed, or even help from a post-natal doula to make the transition out of the new-born time and into babyhood.

But most of all, sleep when your baby sleeps. Take power naps and notice how you feel, and if you can't sleep in the day try instead to lie down and practise awareness of your breath and sensations, or put on a guided relaxation to listen to. Be aware of the quality of your sleep at night. If you find your nervous system is overstimulated from repeated waking, and that you don't settle back to sleep easily, consider finding a naturopath who will be able to advise you on dietary support and appropriate B vitamins and minerals such as magnesium, which are essential for the healthy functioning of the nerves.

Also, carve out a little time each day for exercise. When your body has healed from birth, activities like yoga and Pilates are good for relaxation and helping to strengthen the pelvic floor, while a good walk or even a dance in the living room can be uplifting after a disturbed night. To deepen sleep and release tension, avoid screen use in the evenings and try some stretching, meditation or taking a hot bath before bed. Sleep has a huge impact on our wellness and contentment and it is really worth paying attention to. The more we can improve it, the better we will feel.

BABY

◆

Holding a newborn baby is an extraordinary experience, and the most profound mindfulness meditation we will ever enter into. For a parent in particular, the experience of gazing at their child can far outweigh the beauty of just about anything else in life.

BECOMING A NEW PARENT is an amazing opportunity to lovingly witness the miraculous unfolding and growth of a unique and fresh little being, right from the beginning and all the way through their lives. The exquisite sensitivity and absolute presence that is perceptible in this tiny human form is mesmerizing, and the more conscious we become as we encounter him, the more we can feel into the subtle energy of love and peace that he emanates. These qualities might not be so obvious when a baby is crying, but they are innate.

Bonding

At a subtle level, a mother and her babe will still be connected energetically long after the birth. Even though new babies sleep a lot, they can sense the closeness of their mothers, and many newborns settle much more easily in the support of a sling against their mother's body. It is the most familiar body to them; the sound of the heartbeat and voice, the smell of skin and milk, the warmth and the mother's energy field, are all home to her child. A father or partner's body of course gives similar comfort and familiar vocal sound, and being in the sling is a wonderful way for partners to bond with their baby, especially when it is not possible for a mother to use a sling post-birth.

Being skin-to-skin is also an important part of nurturing a baby, and making special time for this hugely supports the process of bonding for both parents with their newborn. These moments can also become meditations on the sensory experience of being with your baby. Noticing what you see as you behold them, the sensation and warmth of being skin-to-skin, the smell of your baby, the sounds they make, the thoughts and emotions that are evoked in you – all these observations play a part in helping us to become more present and curious about this magical experience.

———————◆———————

There is nothing on earth like the moment
of seeing one's first baby ... there is no height like this
simple one, occurring continuously throughout all ages
in musty bedrooms, in palaces, in caves and desert
places. I looked at this rolled-up bundle and knew again
I had not created her. She was herself apart from me.
She had her own life to lead, her own destiny to
accomplish; she just came past me to this earth.

FROM 'THROUGH MINE OWN EYES'
KATHERINE TREVELYAN

———————◆———————

Wide Awake

Babies are intelligent in a non-intellectual sense; they are delicate, deeply sensitive and receptive to the beings around them. They are also aware in ways we might not realize. I have several specific memories of recognizing that my tiny babies were completely present to my own experience. One was when I was feeling very emotional and crying as I cradled my daughter and she reached her hand up and started patting me in the area of my heart. She was just four months old at that time and had never done this before. I don't know if she had been sleeping, but her timing was immaculate. My son, also, could sense if I was in a bad mood from lack of sleep and, from around four months, would make eye contact with me and then start smiling and giggling, reminding me to enjoy the moment.

These incidents could be explained away as nothings, but as their mother I sensed their significance and knew they showed my children's heightened awareness and engagement in our shared experience. And their intuition can keep growing as they do if we understand and make space for it. I truly believe we can learn so much from our children at all stages of their development and that we should respect and trust in their instinctual wisdom.

Babies are aware in ways
we might not realize

Crying

Crying is one of a baby's primary means of communication and it can happen for many different reasons, from tiredness or hunger to physical pain or needing comfort. It is not always easy to know why your baby is crying or what they need, but as with any student, a parent makes mental notes, responds intuitively, takes guesses, asks a fellow parent and figures things out step by step. Our inbuilt reaction is to soothe a baby when she cries and we will do whatever we can to address the cause of her discomfort.

As someone who sees the benefits of attachment-style parenting, I have confidence that a crying baby can often be comforted by feeding, cuddling and sleep. But there are times when he can't and in instances such as these, he is almost certainly feeling physical discomfort. Unfortunately, all babies experience some degree of pain in their first year of life, through wind trapped temporarily in their tiny bellies, a high fever with teething, etc. Soothing them with our love can help them through it, but no matter how difficult it may be to see them suffering, it is a part of our existence that they become familiar with early on. However, if your baby is in distress and nothing you have tried is working, do take them to see a paediatrician or doctor – even if they fall asleep in the car and it turns out to be nothing, it's still worth the journey. Always take medical advice if this is a common occurrence or if you can't resolve a baby's discomfort and upset.

Coping with Colic

When she was a week or two old, my daughter developed terrible colic, which lasted for over two months and was physically very painful for her and emotionally agonizing for us. Every day, between three and six in the afternoon, she screamed inconsolably in our arms as we tried out every gentle massage, comforting and holding technique we could find to try to ease her sore tummy. Only a small percentage of babies go through colic and there is a lot of information available for parents on causes, symptoms and potential remedies for this condition, which I am not going into here. But if your baby does have colic, it is reassuring to know that it will only last until they are around three months old. This might seem an aeon at the time, but it passes quickly.

ORDINARY CRYING

For first-time parents especially, hearing one's baby cry can create a lot of anxiety, and there can be feelings of awkwardness about this happening in a public place, as though it might reflect some level of inadequacy on our parental capacities. But the truth is that many people are parents themselves and have spent time with crying babies and know it is an ordinary occurrence. Ignoring a distressed child's needs is not something that anyone should condone, but attending to an upset baby is just a part of parental life and is not something to feel embarrassed about around others.

On the other hand, coping strategies for parents of colicky or frequently crying babies are also important, because this can be a harrowing experience and whoever is caring for the baby while they are crying needs to be able to manage and regulate their own state of being. It can help to practise mindful breathing and to try to relax as much as possible while comforting your little one. Also, become consciously aware of any fears or negative thoughts and just name them one by one as they arise. Try to welcome your feelings without needing to change them, but continue relaxing with your breath if you can; if you can't, try counting to four as you inhale and again as you exhale, to focus your mind.

It's good to know when you need a break and to swap with your partner at those times. If you are alone, do whatever helps you to release tension, even if that means putting your baby down for a few minutes, making sure they are safe, and taking some deep breaths in the next room; or putting on some music, or going out for a walk with your baby in the sling in the hope that they might find relaxation in the rhythm of walking and fall asleep.

ON BEING A FATHER OR PARTNER

◆

You are a father. I honour you. By embodying this role, you become an irreplaceable, powerful, loving presence in your child's life, a beloved parent and partner within your family. Be proud of walking the path of fatherhood, because it is an amazing route to take.

For a father or partner, adjusting to family life with a new baby may bring the sense of being a scaffold that supports this delicate mother-baby dyad and perhaps other children, too. This can catalyse combinations of differing responses, from feeling needed and loved to feeling like you need to be a hero, to feeling excluded, to fear of responsibility, intimacy or sleep deprivation. You may be in a blissful state of connection and falling in love with your baby, but there might also be a complex array of other inner experiences at play. And it can be both a beautiful and an emotional time, depending on your family's experience of childbirth, of post-birth and on how much support you have around you.

Remembering the human-ness in your situation is of great value. Firstly, that you are only able to do and give what you can, as a human being. Help as much as possible, but don't overstretch yourself without topping up on what nourishes you and keeps you smiling. Secondly, in recognizing the human frailty of the newborn time, that everyone will be doing their best to keep on keeping on, including your baby,

---

For the majority of mothers, a most
important ingredient for her successful pregnancy,
birth and breastfeeding is the quality of care
she receives from the father.

FROM 'FATHERS-TO-BE HANDBOOK'
PATRICK M. HOUSER

---

and that both patience and compassion are required to *be* with
all the sides of your life right now, just as they are, which may
in some cases be 'unsolvable' or beyond your control.

Support Yourself

Keep encouraging yourself, too. Your support is vital to your
family – even if it sometimes looks like you are an outsider
to your partner and child, you are actually an invaluable
co-member of their world and they need you. But consider
the following areas to support yourself too. These are actually
relevant to both parents at different stages:

• **Sleep** If you are not well enough rested, this can take a toll
on your overall well-being and immune system. Think about
ways to improve your quantity and quality of sleep when you
are not helping out on a night shift. Try using earplugs, sleeping
in another room, avoiding caffeine, drinking less fluids in the
evening to avoid urinating in the night. Before bed, try yoga,
meditation or taking a hot bath.

- **Exercise** Call it raising the endorphins or letting off steam, regular exercise is crucial for restoring the mind and body to balance and helping us to unwind, especially if our nerves are edgy from lack of sleep. Even if sport or going to the gym isn't your thing, go for a long run or walk, dance, box, cycle or swim, even try energetic vacuuming, or whatever it takes to bring you into a place of harmony.

- **Enjoyment** Take a bit of time every week or so to do something you love, just for you. Creating a window of space that is *your* time, like a fun reward, will help to make the time dedicated to your family feel less dutiful (if that is how it's been), fresher and more heartfelt.

- **Meditation** Although having a regular meditation practice requires discipline, its benefits are beyond measure and they will fortify your parenting abilities in every way. For both parents, meditating is also a valuable way of inwardly managing the effects of a traumatic birth experience and it is worth setting aside the time if this has been the case for you. But even if not, you will still no doubt notice the positive effects of just five or ten minutes of sitting mindfulness practice, morning and evening. If you can't manage this daily, even trying to fit in a few moments, a few breaths, here and there when you remember, will help too.

Being lovers is still important
for the joy of your connection

Partnership

If this is your first child, you may feel that the overnight transition from being lovers to being parents can be a bit of a shock. A new kind of love dawns in your relationship that involves inordinate amounts of giving to a very small person. A love that is not specifically about being two lovers in the traditional sense, but one that grows your hearts beyond this terminology. However, being lovers is still important for the joy of your connection and the health of your relationship, and eventually it will need to thrive in balance with parenting, but to begin with it takes second place because your baby's needs naturally come first.

A mother will usually be utterly aware of this fact and, in some ways, it is actually the father or partner who needs to consciously adjust their perception and expectations of their partnership to accommodate the new family dynamics. But this might be easier said than done and it could leave grey areas of assumption, misunderstanding and unexpressed feelings unless both parents make the space to express any hidden issues going on internally.

Communication

If you are feeling uneasy about something between you and your partner, I would invite you to take a few minutes for yourself, to reflect on what your feelings are and where they are coming from. If you find that they hold some weight and are not just passing irritations or momentary blips, the next step is to communicate these feelings clearly. Speaking honestly can sometimes be unsettling or upsetting, and for fathers and partners it is wise to tread carefully with a new mother as she will probably be feeling both emotionally and physically sensitive after the birth. Nevertheless, holding back your emotions only escalates them. If you can find a way to calmly bare your heart and be honestly vulnerable, without blame or drama, taking full responsibility for your feelings, your partner will most probably be open to hearing you.

Here, trust comes into its own, firstly as an overriding vehicle for the belief that you can still be lovers even when you are parents, but know that flexibility and patience will be needed. And secondly in our sharing – if we can communicate with the trust that we will be loved and heard, we can allow ourselves to be real and vulnerable in our relationship together. Everything that fosters trust between partners and within a family is significant and this can start very simply with the way we speak to each other. It's a great idea to practise communicating with kindness before babies and children arrive, but it is never too late to learn if you have them already, and it can only improve your relationships and interactions with those you love. (See resources section for more ideas.)

PARENTHOOD

◆

The act of bearing children connects us both to our ancestral past and to future generations, and as we become a living link in the vast chain of human lives, it might dawn on us that this is one of the most important things we will ever do.

BEING A PARENT SOMETIMES CAUSES us to touch into the extremes of our hearts. It is as humbling a task as one that may make us proud, and it can be as joyful as it is difficult at times. In the quiet moments you have spare, just check in with your feelings about your life with a new baby. They may be diverse and even contradictory, but try to welcome them all, even if you have judgements about some. Give time to acknowledge each of your feelings as perfect expressions of where you are at this point in your life, knowing that this post-birth time is a period of integration. By integration, I mean the conscious or unconscious process of meeting and reconciling ourselves with our living reality.

You could say that life itself is one long process of integration, which it is in a way, but it is particularly applicable to big life events, like the initial stage of birthing and parenting a baby, which presents such a huge shift in parents' lives – because in this situation we find both enjoyable and uneasy reactions in ourselves that we might not have expected. We encounter the light and the shadow in our own psyche and in our experiences and we must somehow find confluence with them from day to day, even when it is uncomfortable.

Perfect but Not Faultless

I remember believing that I would be a 'perfect parent', that I would do everything right and never raise my voice to my children, and that anything less than this would really not be good enough. And right from their babyhood I did try very hard to achieve these goals, to always respond with love and to give of myself whatever my children required. But in so doing I set myself up for failure, because the pressure to do everything 'right' brought heaviness and self-judgement into my being. I tried too hard and ended up punishing myself for what I felt to be my shortcomings. If I was agitated because my sleep was being disrupted, I felt I had failed.

The mature heart is not perfectionistic:
it rests in compassion for our being instead of in ideals
of the mind ... Mature spirituality is not based on
seeking perfection, on achieving some imaginary sense
of purity. It is based on the capacity to let go and to
love, to open the heart to all that is.

FROM 'BRINGING HOME THE DHARMA'
JACK KORNFIELD

Meditation was the best tool I had to integrate my experiences of failure with my deeper feeling that I was actually doing my best. As my children grew, I was able to ground myself in a daily practice of sitting in that place between the play of the mind and pure presence, just observing the dance between them and discovering a compassionate centre within me, encompassing all. It was through this practice, and the parenting of my children, that I learned how to start healing and to embrace myself, without apology, showing up as I am for them on good days and hard ones. The reality remains that I am the perfect parent for my children, but that does not mean I am perfect in the sense of being faultless.

A Transformative Experience

So parenthood has been a wholly transformative experience for me and I believe it can be like this for many of us when we walk mindfully on the path. If we can continue to offer ourselves compassion, however we are feeling, the process flows more easily, even in the face of challenges. It can take time, but there will be a deeper current of integration happening and by bringing mindful awareness to our feelings and related thoughts, we can assist it.

But like any process of creation, making a family requires inner adjustments and a lot of learning, and the course will not always run smooth. Sometimes our needs will not be met by another, or by our circumstances, and there will also be times when we are unable to fulfil the wishes or requirements of our family members. Here we may encounter our own feelings of disappointment and failure. But in trying to approach parenthood with a sense of acceptance for what is, and for how we are, we can hold the light and the dark, the sunny and the stormy aspects within ourselves more in balance. Because these are the qualities that work together to integrate us as people, and when we can own and appreciate both, we are free to be ourselves authentically.

Domestic Bliss

When you have a baby, it is a good idea to lower the standards in your living environment and yet celebrate your efforts for everything you do each day, even if that means that the house is chaos, with dishes unwashed and floors unswept. If cooking feels like an extra demand, then try eating simple, nutritious and easy food, while putting minimal effort into preparing it. I once met a wonderful mother with twins whom I questioned about how she managed to meet everyone's needs and

---

I can lose myself and find myself simultaneously while cleaning the kitchen stove. This is a great, if rare occasion for mindfulness practice.

FROM 'WHEREVER YOU GO, THERE YOU ARE'
JON KABAT-ZINN

MINDFUL PRACTICE FOR DOMESTIC CHORES

Sit or stand quietly in the area you want to clean. Close your eyes and become aware of the flow of your breath in and out.

- Notice how your body feels right now and let yourself relax a little more.
- Then open your eyes and with a gentle gaze, just scan the living space around you.
- Observe the commentary that comes up for you about what you are seeing. If there are judgements or perhaps a sense of urgency to improve it all, keep these in your awareness without reacting to them.
- When you are ready, calmly approach your chore in a mindful state, keeping your attention with the task at hand as much as possible.
- If you notice your mind wandering, just return to the present moment and to your breath, with acceptance.
- See if you can continue whatever it is you are doing and find some joy in the movement, the physical sensations, in all that you can see, hear and experience.

When you have finished the chore, pause for a moment to recognize your efforts, and breathe.

she smiled, then laughed and said, 'Well, we have very low expectations!' For me, this is the perfect maxim for early parenthood and it brings elements of mindfulness, such as patience and just meeting life as it is, into daily practice.

As long as you and your baby are happy and healthy, whatever else you are doing is enough. If you find you are careworn or stressed by your home and lifestyle being turned upside down, just feel into those edges of your comfort zone and try to relax and practise some compassion for yourself. What you are doing is not easy and it is worthy of patience. In years to come things will change, but for now simply acknowledge all that you *are* doing and know that you deserve kindness. From this compassionate place, everything will feel easier, but this exercise may help at those opportune moments when you do want to wrestle with the dust.

As Time Goes By

The idea of gradually 'returning to normal' when you have a new addition to the family is a peculiar one – because firstly, is there ever a normal in this ever-changing, cycling of life that we are ensconced in? And secondly, whatever 'normal' we may have known rapidly becomes a new normal, which will really keep us on our toes, because it too will be changing so fast with the growth and development of this little baby. Expect change, and try to embrace it. In terms of living life mindfully, children ask that we stay open to who they keep becoming, from week to week and year to year. They are our guides and taskmasters, engaging our curiosity with their own, proving to us that life is one big adventure into transition after transition, and that holding back will only disconnect us from its flow.

Life with children is an experiential meditation practice on the impermanent nature of existence and in this respect, and many others, it is a spiritual path. I still come across photos and video clips of my kids from time to time and long to cuddle them as little ones again, but I try to just feel into my longing and my breath, knowing that this too will change. Looking back like this also enables me to recognize the importance of finding the joy and beauty even in mundane aspects of life, because it moves so quickly – and if we miss this, here and now, we lose the opportunity to really receive it.

All we need to remember is to receive the present.

Your children are not your children.
They are the sons and daughters of Life's
longing for itself …
For life goes not backward nor tarries with yesterday.
You are the bows from which your children
as living arrows are sent forth.

FROM 'THE PROPHET'
KAHLIL GIBRAN (1883–1931)

RESOURCES

◆

Pregnancy reading for parents

Gentle Birth, Gentle Mothering, Sarah Buckley (Celestial Arts, 2009)
Ina May's Guide to Childbirth, Ina May Gaskin (Bantam Dell, 2003)
Mindful Birthing, Nancy Bardacke (Harper Collins, 2012)
Childbirth Without Fear, Grantly Dick-Read (Pinter & Martin, 2013)
Water, Birth & Sexuality, Michel Odent (Clairview Books, 2014)
Men, Love & Birth, Mark Harris (Pinter & Martin, 2015)
Fathers-To-Be, Patrick M. Houser (Creative Life Systems, 2007)

Doula organizations

DOULA UK: www.doula.org.uk
EDN: European-doula-network.org
DONA INTERNATIONAL: www.dona.org
AUSTRALIAN DOULAS: www.australiandoulas.com.au

Birth links

BIRTH POSITIONS: *New Active Birth*, Janet Balaskas (Thorsons, 1990),
activebirthcentre.com
ACUPRESSURE: Debra Betts – acupressure in childbirth, acupuncture.rhizome.net.nz
To download her free booklet, visit acupuncture.rhizome.net.nz/download-booklet/
REBOZO SHAWL TECHNIQUES: spinningbabies.com, and doulas trained by Traditional
Mexican midwife Angelina Martinez
BIRTH PREFERENCES TEMPLATES: www.lamaze.org; www.nct.org.uk
GENTLE CAESAREAN BIRTH PLANS: www.motherlove.com/blog/view/
Writing-a-family-centred-caesarean-birth-plan, www.birthwithoutfearblog.com
SEEDING A BABY'S MICROBIOME AT BIRTH: *The Microbiome Effect* by Toni Harman and
Alex Wakeford (Pinter & Martin, 2016). Documentary film 'Microbirth' at
www.microbirth.com
GOLDEN HOUR: choicesinchildbirth.org; www.perinatalnetwork.org;
www.bellybelly.com.au; magicalhour.com

Breastfeeding

Ina May's Guide to Breastfeeding, Ina May Gaskin (Pinter & Martin, 2009)
The Womanly Art of Breastfeeding, La Leche League International
(Pinter & Martin, 2010)
The Food of Love, Kate Evans (Myriad Editions, 2008)

Breastfeeding support organizations

UK: www.tongue-tie.org.uk; www.abm.me.uk; www.laleche.org.uk;
www.breastfeedingnetwork.org.uk; www.nct.org.uk;
www.nationalbreastfeedinghelpline.org.uk;
USA: www.lllusa.org; www.pebblesofhope.org; www.mhpsalud.org/Breastfeeding;
www.breastfeedingusa.org; www.naba-breastfeeding.org
INTERNATIONAL: www.llli.org; www.breastfeeding.asn.au;
www.lalecheleague.org.nz; www.babyfriendly.org.nz; www.waba.org.my
FOR MULTIPLE BIRTHS: www.raisingmultiples.org;
www.tamba.org.uk/Parent-Support

Post-birth

POSTNATAL DEPRESSION SUPPORT ORGANIZATIONS:
UK: www.mothersformothers.co.uk; www.pandasfoundation.org.uk;
www.nct.org.uk; www.pni.org.uk; www.bestbeginnings.org.uk
USA: www.postpartum.net; www.crisistextline.org;
www.maternalmentalhealthnow.org
INTERNATIONAL: www.panda.org.au; www.pnd.org.nz; www.mentalhealth.org;
www.mentalhealth.org.nz
FATHERS-TO-BE: www.fatherstobe.org
MEAL PLANNER FOR FRIENDS AND RELATIVES TO PAMPER YOU POST-BIRTH:
www.takethemameal.com

Further reading

When Survivors Give Birth, Penny Simkin & Phyllis Klaus (Classic Day Publishing, 2004)
NVC — Nonviolent Communication: A Language of Life, Marshal B. Rosenberg and Arun Gandhi (Puddledancer Press, 2015)
Parent Effectiveness Training, Thomas Gordon (Three Rivers Press, 2008)
The Gifts of Imperfect Parenting Audio CD by Brené Brown (Sounds True, 2013)
Finding Your Inner Mama edited by Eden Steinberg (Shambhala, 2007)
Zen & the Path of Mindful Parenting, Clea Danaan (Leaping Hare Press, 2015)
Bringing Home the Dharma, Jack Kornfield (Shambhala, 2012)
Magical Beginnings, Enchanted Lives, Deepak Chopra (Crown Publications, 2005)
Wherever You Go, There You Are, Jon Kabat-Zinn (Piatkus, 2004)
Through Mine Own Eyes, Katherine Trevelyan (Kessinger Publishing, 2010)
Ten Moons — The Inner Journey of Pregnancy, Jane Hardwicke Collings (Lulu Publishing, 2016)

INDEX

INDEX

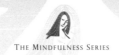

THE MINDFULNESS SERIES

DEDICATION & ACKNOWLEDGEMENTS

I dedicate this book to my beloved children,
Anoushka and Orlando, and to all children.

With deepest gratitude to my amazing husband, Robin,
for all his love and support; to my parents and my brother;
to my women's circle of dear friends; to Kate Woods and all of my doula
colleagues; to Janet Balaskas; and finally to Susan, Monica, Joanna and Jenni
at Leaping Hare Press for helping me to birth this book into being.

Visit rigaforbes.co.uk to download free audio recordings of exercises in this book.

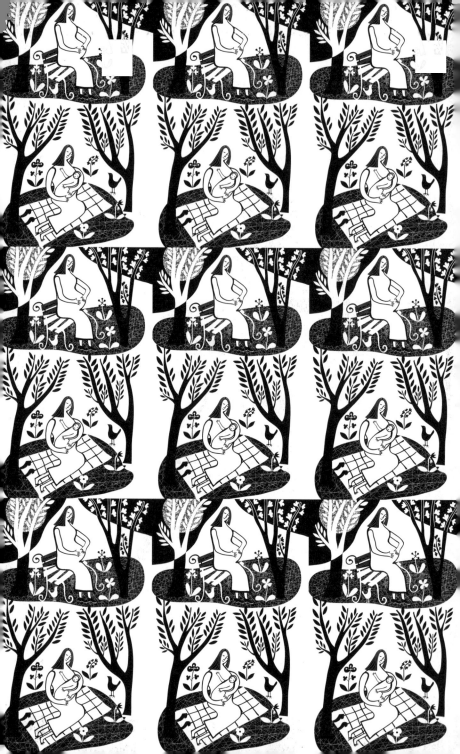